Workout Log

by
Ed Alicea

Bloomington, IN Milton Keynes, UK

authorHOUSE

AuthorHouse™
1663 Liberty Drive, Suite 200
Bloomington, IN 47403
www.authorhouse.com
Phone: 1-800-839-8640

AuthorHouse™ UK Ltd.
500 Avebury Boulevard
Central Milton Keynes, MK9 2BE
www.authorhouse.co.uk
Phone: 08001974150

First published by AuthorHouse 7/27/2006

ISBN: 1-4208-9536-2 (sc)

*Printed in the United States of America
Bloomington, Indiana*

This book is printed on acid-free paper.

How to use this log

Use this log to track your progress and help you reach your individual goals from workout to workout and meal to meal.

Exercise Section:

Simply record the amount of weight lifted and the number of repetitions for each exercise.

Meal Section:

Record your calories, carbs, protein, fat, and sodium intake for each meal and time of meal up to 5 times per day.

Measurement Section:

Included at the beginning and the end of this 3 month planner is the measurement page, to record your measurements for each body part and your total weight.

Remember:

Tracking your exercise and meal is one of the keys to fitness success.

Measurements

Neck   _____

Arms   _____

Chest   _____

Waist   _____

Hips   _____

Thighs   _____

Calves   _____

Weight   _____

EXERCISE PLANNER

Sunday_____   Month_____   Yr___

Exercise_____   **Exercise**_____   **Exercise**_____

   Weight   Reps   Weight   Reps   Weight   Reps

1.   X   1.   X   1.   X
2.   X   2.   X   2.   X
3.   X   3.   X   3.   X
4.   X   4.   X   4.   X
5.   X   5.   X   5.   X

Exercise_____   **Exercise**_____   **Exercise**_____

   Weight   Reps   Weight   Reps   Weight   Reps

1.   X   1.   X   1.   X
2.   X   2.   X   2.   X
3.   X   3.   X   3.   X
4.   X   4.   X   4.   X
5.   X   5.   X   5.   X

Exercise_____   **Exercise**_____   **Exercise**_____

   Weight   Reps   Weight   Reps   Weight   Reps

1.   X   1.   X   1.   X
2.   X   2.   X   2.   X
3.   X   3.   X   3.   X
4.   X   4.   X   4.   X
5.   X   5.   X   5.   X

Exercise_____   **Exercise**_____   **Exercise**_____

   Weight   Reps   Weight   Reps   Weight   Reps

1.   X   1.   X   1.   X
2.   X   2.   X   2.   X
3.   X   3.   X   3.   X
4.   X   4.   X   4.   X
5.   X   5.   X   5.   X

Aerobic Workout   **ABS**

Exercise   Time   Exercise_____

1._____   ____Min/Hr Set/Reps 1.____   2.____   3.____

2._____   ____Min/Hr Exercise_____

                             Set/Reps 1.____   2.____   3.____

Monday_____   Month_____ Yr___

Exercise_____   **Exercise_____**   **Exercise_____**

   Weight   Reps   Weight   Reps   Weight   Reps

1.   X   1.   X   1.   X
2.   X   2.   X   2.   X
3.   X   3.   X   3.   X
4.   X   4.   X   4.   X
5.   X   5.   X   5.   X

Exercise_____   **Exercise_____**   **Exercise_____**

   Weight   Reps   Weight   Reps   Weight   Reps

1.   X   1.   X   1.   X
2.   X   2.   X   2.   X
3.   X   3.   X   3.   X
4.   X   4.   X   4.   X
5.   X   5.   X   5.   X

Exercise_____   **Exercise_____**   **Exercise_____**

   Weight   Reps   Weight   Reps   Weight   Reps

1.   X   1.   X   1.   X
2.   X   2.   X   2.   X
3.   X   3.   X   3.   X
4.   X   4.   X   4.   X
5.   X   5.   X   5.   X

Exercise_____   **Exercise_____**   **Exercise_____**

   Weight   Reps   Weight   Reps   Weight   Reps

1.   X   1.   X   1.   X
2.   X   2.   X   2.   X
3.   X   3.   X   3.   X
4.   X   4.   X   4.   X
5.   X   5.   X   5.   X

Aerobic Workout   **ABS**

Exercise   Time   Exercise_____

1._____   ____Min/Hr   Set/Reps 1._____   2._____   3._____

2._____   ____Min/Hr   Exercise_____

                                 Set/Reps 1._____   2._____   3._____

3

Tuesday_____   Month_____ Yr___

Exercise_____   **Exercise**_____   **Exercise**_____

   Weight   Reps   Weight   Reps   Weight   Reps

1.   X   1.   X   1.   X
2.   X   2.   X   2.   X
3.   X   3.   X   3.   X
4.   X   4.   X   4.   X
5.   X   5.   X   5.   X

Exercise_____   **Exercise**_____   **Exercise**_____

   Weight   Reps   Weight   Reps   Weight   Reps

1.   X   1.   X   1.   X
2.   X   2.   X   2.   X
3.   X   3.   X   3.   X
4.   X   4.   X   4.   X
5.   X   5.   X   5.   X

Exercise_____   **Exercise**_____   **Exercise**_____

   Weight   Reps   Weight   Reps   Weight   Reps

1.   X   1.   X   1.   X
2.   X   2.   X   2.   X
3.   X   3.   X   3.   X
4.   X   4.   X   4.   X
5.   X   5.   X   5.   X

Exercise_____   **Exercise**_____   **Exercise**_____

   Weight   Reps   Weight   Reps   Weight   Reps

1.   X   1.   X   1.   X
2.   X   2.   X   2.   X
3.   X   3.   X   3.   X
4.   X   4.   X   4.   X
5.   X   5.   X   5.   X

Aerobic Workout   **ABS**

Exercise   Time   Exercise_____

1._____   ____Min/Hr Set/Reps 1.____   2.____   3.____

2._____   ____Min/Hr Exercise_____

                              Set/Reps 1.____   2.____   3.____

Wednesday_____   Month_____ Yr___

Exercise_____   **Exercise_____**   **Exercise_____**

    Weight   Reps   Weight   Reps   Weight   Reps

1.   X   1.   X   1.   X
2.   X   2.   X   2.   X
3.   X   3.   X   3.   X
4.   X   4.   X   4.   X
5.   X   5.   X   5.   X

Exercise_____   **Exercise_____**   **Exercise_____**

    Weight   Reps   Weight   Reps   Weight   Reps

1.   X   1.   X   1.   X
2.   X   2.   X   2.   X
3.   X   3.   X   3.   X
4.   X   4.   X   4.   X
5.   X   5.   X   5.   X

Exercise_____   **Exercise_____**   **Exercise_____**

    Weight   Reps   Weight   Reps   Weight   Reps

1.   X   1.   X   1.   X
2.   X   2.   X   2.   X
3.   X   3.   X   3.   X
4.   X   4.   X   4.   X
5.   X   5.   X   5.   X

Exercise_____   **Exercise_____**   **Exercise_____**

    Weight   Reps   Weight   Reps   Weight   Reps

1.   X   1.   X   1.   X
2.   X   2.   X   2.   X
3.   X   3.   X   3.   X
4.   X   4.   X   4.   X
5.   X   5.   X   5.   X

Aerobic Workout   **ABS**

Exercise   Time   Exercise_____

1._____   ____Min/Hr Set/Reps 1.____   2.____   3.____

2._____   ____Min/Hr Exercise_____

                                Set/Reps 1.____   2.____   3.____

Thursday_____   Month_____ Yr___

Exercise_____   **Exercise_____**   **Exercise_____**

	Weight	Reps			Weight	Reps			Weight	Reps

Weight   Reps   Weight   Reps   Weight   Reps

1.   X   1.   X   1.   X
2.   X   2.   X   2.   X
3.   X   3.   X   3.   X
4.   X   4.   X   4.   X
5.   X   5.   X   5.   X

Exercise_____   **Exercise_____**   **Exercise_____**

Weight   Reps   Weight   Reps   Weight   Reps

1.   X   1.   X   1.   X
2.   X   2.   X   2.   X
3.   X   3.   X   3.   X
4.   X   4.   X   4.   X
5.   X   5.   X   5.   X

Exercise_____   **Exercise_____**   **Exercise_____**

Weight   Reps   Weight   Reps   Weight   Reps

1.   X   1.   X   1.   X
2.   X   2.   X   2.   X
3.   X   3.   X   3.   X
4.   X   4.   X   4.   X
5.   X   5.   X   5.   X

Exercise_____   **Exercise_____**   **Exercise_____**

Weight   Reps   Weight   Reps   Weight   Reps

1.   X   1.   X   1.   X
2.   X   2.   X   2.   X
3.   X   3.   X   3.   X
4.   X   4.   X   4.   X
5.   X   5.   X   5.   X

Aerobic Workout   **ABS**

Exercise   Time   Exercise_____

1._____   ____Min/Hr   Set/Reps   1.____   2.____   3.____

2._____   ____Min/Hr   Exercise_____

                              Set/Reps   1.____   2.____   3.____

Friday_____   Month_____ Yr___

Exercise_____   **Exercise**_____   **Exercise**_____

   Weight   Reps   Weight   Reps   Weight   Reps

1.   X   1.   X   1.   X
2.   X   2.   X   2.   X
3.   X   3.   X   3.   X
4.   X   4.   X   4.   X
5.   X   5.   X   5.   X

Exercise_____   **Exercise**_____   **Exercise**_____

   Weight   Reps   Weight   Reps   Weight   Reps

1.   X   1.   X   1.   X
2.   X   2.   X   2.   X
3.   X   3.   X   3.   X
4.   X   4.   X   4.   X
5.   X   5.   X   5.   X

Exercise_____   **Exercise**_____   **Exercise**_____

   Weight   Reps   Weight   Reps   Weight   Reps

1.   X   1.   X   1.   X
2.   X   2.   X   2.   X
3.   X   3.   X   3.   X
4.   X   4.   X   4.   X
5.   X   5.   X   5.   X

Exercise_____   **Exercise**_____   **Exercise**_____

   Weight   Reps   Weight   Reps   Weight   Reps

1.   X   1.   X   1.   X
2.   X   2.   X   2.   X
3.   X   3.   X   3.   X
4.   X   4.   X   4.   X
5.   X   5.   X   5.   X

Aerobic Workout   **ABS**

Exercise   Time   Exercise_____

1._____   ____Min/Hr Set/Reps 1.____   2.____   3.____

2._____   ____Min/Hr Exercise_____

                             Set/Reps 1.____   2.____   3.____

Saturday_____   Month_____ Yr___

Exercise_____   **Exercise**_____   **Exercise**_____

    Weight   Reps   Weight   Reps   Weight   Reps

1.	X		1.	X		1.	X
2.	X		2.	X		2.	X
3.	X		3.	X		3.	X
4.	X		4.	X		4.	X
5.	X		5.	X		5.	X

Exercise_____   **Exercise**_____   **Exercise**_____

    Weight   Reps   Weight   Reps   Weight   Reps

1.	X		1.	X		1.	X
2.	X		2.	X		2.	X
3.	X		3.	X		3.	X
4.	X		4.	X		4.	X
5.	X		5.	X		5.	X

Exercise_____   **Exercise**_____   **Exercise**_____

    Weight   Reps   Weight   Reps   Weight   Reps

1.	X		1.	X		1.	X
2.	X		2.	X		2.	X
3.	X		3.	X		3.	X
4.	X		4.	X		4.	X
5.	X		5.	X		5.	X

Exercise_____   **Exercise**_____   **Exercise**_____

    Weight   Reps   Weight   Reps   Weight   Reps

1.	X		1.	X		1.	X
2.	X		2.	X		2.	X
3.	X		3.	X		3.	X
4.	X		4.	X		4.	X
5.	X		5.	X		5.	X

Aerobic Workout   **ABS**

Exercise   Time   Exercise_____

1._____ ____Min/Hr   Set/Reps 1.____ 2.____   3.____

2._____ ____Min/Hr   Exercise_____

                        Set/Reps 1.____ 2.____   3.____

8

Notes

Sunday_____   Month_____   Yr___

Exercise_____   **Exercise_____**   **Exercise_____**

  Weight   Reps   Weight   Reps   Weight   Reps

1.   X   1.   X   1.   X
2.   X   2.   X   2.   X
3.   X   3.   X   3.   X
4.   X   4.   X   4.   X
5.   X   5.   X   5.   X

Exercise_____   **Exercise_____**   **Exercise_____**

  Weight   Reps   Weight   Reps   Weight   Reps

1.   X   1.   X   1.   X
2.   X   2.   X   2.   X
3.   X   3.   X   3.   X
4.   X   4.   X   4.   X
5.   X   5.   X   5.   X

Exercise_____   **Exercise_____**   **Exercise_____**

  Weight   Reps   Weight   Reps   Weight   Reps

1.   X   1.   X   1.   X
2.   X   2.   X   2.   X
3.   X   3.   X   3.   X
4.   X   4.   X   4.   X
5.   X   5.   X   5.   X

Exercise_____   **Exercise_____**   **Exercise_____**

  Weight   Reps   Weight   Reps   Weight   Reps

1.   X   1.   X   1.   X
2.   X   2.   X   2.   X
3.   X   3.   X   3.   X
4.   X   4.   X   4.   X
5.   X   5.   X   5.   X

Aerobic Workout   **ABS**

Exercise   Time   Exercise_____

1._____   ____Min/Hr Set/Reps 1.____   2.____   3.____

2._____   ____Min/Hr Exercise_____

                              Set/Reps 1.____   2.____   3.____

Monday_____   Month____ Yr___

Exercise_____   **Exercise_____**   **Exercise_____**

   Weight   Reps   Weight   Reps   Weight   Reps

1.   X   1.   X   1.   X
2.   X   2.   X   2.   X
3.   X   3.   X   3.   X
4.   X   4.   X   4.   X
5.   X   5.   X   5.   X

Exercise_____   **Exercise_____**   **Exercise_____**

   Weight   Reps   Weight   Reps   Weight   Reps

1.   X   1.   X   1.   X
2.   X   2.   X   2.   X
3.   X   3.   X   3.   X
4.   X   4.   X   4.   X
5.   X   5.   X   5.   X

Exercise_____   **Exercise_____**   **Exercise_____**

   Weight   Reps   Weight   Reps   Weight   Reps

1.   X   1.   X   1.   X
2.   X   2.   X   2.   X
3.   X   3.   X   3.   X
4.   X   4.   X   4.   X
5.   X   5.   X   5.   X

Exercise_____   **Exercise_____**   **Exercise_____**

   Weight   Reps   Weight   Reps   Weight   Reps

1.   X   1.   X   1.   X
2.   X   2.   X   2.   X
3.   X   3.   X   3.   X
4.   X   4.   X   4.   X
5.   X   5.   X   5.   X

Aerobic Workout   **ABS**

Exercise   Time   Exercise_____

1._____   ____Min/Hr Set/Reps 1.____   2.____   3.____

2._____   ____Min/Hr Exercise_____

                               Set/Reps 1.____   2.____   3.____

Tuesday_____   Month_____ Yr____

Exercise_____   **Exercise_____**   **Exercise_____**

   Weight   Reps   Weight   Reps   Weight   Reps

1.   X   1.   X   1.   X
2.   X   2.   X   2.   X
3.   X   3.   X   3.   X
4.   X   4.   X   4.   X
5.   X   5.   X   5.   X

Exercise_____   **Exercise_____**   **Exercise_____**

   Weight   Reps   Weight   Reps   Weight   Reps

1.   X   1.   X   1.   X
2.   X   2.   X   2.   X
3.   X   3.   X   3.   X
4.   X   4.   X   4.   X
5.   X   5.   X   5.   X

Exercise_____   **Exercise_____**   **Exercise_____**

   Weight   Reps   Weight   Reps   Weight   Reps

1.   X   1.   X   1.   X
2.   X   2.   X   2.   X
3.   X   3.   X   3.   X
4.   X   4.   X   4.   X
5.   X   5.   X   5.   X

Exercise_____   **Exercise_____**   **Exercise_____**

   Weight   Reps   Weight   Reps   Weight   Reps

1.   X   1.   X   1.   X
2.   X   2.   X   2.   X
3.   X   3.   X   3.   X
4.   X   4.   X   4.   X
5.   X   5.   X   5.   X

Aerobic Workout   **ABS**

Exercise   Time   Exercise_____

1._____   ____Min/Hr Set/Reps 1.____   2.____   3.____

2._____   ____Min/Hr Exercise_____

                              Set/Reps 1.____   2.____   3.____

Wednesday_____   Month_____ Yr___

Exercise_____   **Exercise_____**   **Exercise_____**

   Weight   Reps   Weight   Reps   Weight   Reps

1.   X   1.   X   1.   X
2.   X   2.   X   2.   X
3.   X   3.   X   3.   X
4.   X   4.   X   4.   X
5.   X   5.   X   5.   X

Exercise_____   **Exercise_____**   **Exercise_____**

   Weight   Reps   Weight   Reps   Weight   Reps

1.   X   1.   X   1.   X
2.   X   2.   X   2.   X
3.   X   3.   X   3.   X
4.   X   4.   X   4.   X
5.   X   5.   X   5.   X

Exercise_____   **Exercise_____**   **Exercise_____**

   Weight   Reps   Weight   Reps   Weight   Reps

1.   X   1.   X   1.   X
2.   X   2.   X   2.   X
3.   X   3.   X   3.   X
4.   X   4.   X   4.   X
5.   X   5.   X   5.   X

Exercise_____   **Exercise_____**   **Exercise_____**

   Weight   Reps   Weight   Reps   Weight   Reps

1.   X   1.   X   1.   X
2.   X   2.   X   2.   X
3.   X   3.   X   3.   X
4.   X   4.   X   4.   X
5.   X   5.   X   5.   X

Aerobic Workout   **ABS**

Exercise   Time   Exercise_____

1._____ ____Min/Hr Set/Reps 1.____ 2.____ 3.____

2._____ ____Min/Hr Exercise_____

                       Set/Reps 1.____ 2.____ 3.____

Thursday_____   Month_____ Yr___

Exercise_____ **Exercise**_____ **Exercise**_____

    Weight   Reps   Weight   Reps   Weight   Reps

1.   X   1.   X   1.   X
2.   X   2.   X   2.   X
3.   X   3.   X   3.   X
4.   X   4.   X   4.   X
5.   X   5.   X   5.   X

Exercise_____ **Exercise**_____ **Exercise**_____

    Weight   Reps   Weight   Reps   Weight   Reps

1.   X   1.   X   1.   X
2.   X   2.   X   2.   X
3.   X   3.   X   3.   X
4.   X   4.   X   4.   X
5.   X   5.   X   5.   X

Exercise_____ **Exercise**_____ **Exercise**_____

    Weight   Reps   Weight   Reps   Weight   Reps

1.   X   1.   X   1.   X
2.   X   2.   X   2.   X
3.   X   3.   X   3.   X
4.   X   4.   X   4.   X
5.   X   5.   X   5.   X

Exercise_____ **Exercise**_____ **Exercise**_____

    Weight   Reps   Weight   Reps   Weight   Reps

1.   X   1.   X   1.   X
2.   X   2.   X   2.   X
3.   X   3.   X   3.   X
4.   X   4.   X   4.   X
5.   X   5.   X   5.   X

Aerobic Workout   **ABS**

Exercise   Time   Exercise_____

1._____   ____Min/Hr Set/Reps 1.____ 2.____   3.____

2._____   ____Min/Hr Exercise_____

                            Set/Reps 1.____ 2.____   3.____

Friday_____   Month_____ Yr___

Exercise_____   **Exercise_____**   **Exercise_____**

   Weight   Reps   Weight   Reps   Weight   Reps

1.   X   1.   X   1.   X
2.   X   2.   X   2.   X
3.   X   3.   X   3.   X
4.   X   4.   X   4.   X
5.   X   5.   X   5.   X

Exercise_____   **Exercise_____**   **Exercise_____**

   Weight   Reps   Weight   Reps   Weight   Reps

1.   X   1.   X   1.   X
2.   X   2.   X   2.   X
3.   X   3.   X   3.   X
4.   X   4.   X   4.   X
5.   X   5.   X   5.   X

Exercise_____   **Exercise_____**   **Exercise_____**

   Weight   Reps   Weight   Reps   Weight   Reps

1.   X   1.   X   1.   X
2.   X   2.   X   2.   X
3.   X   3.   X   3.   X
4.   X   4.   X   4.   X
5.   X   5.   X   5.   X

Exercise_____   **Exercise_____**   **Exercise_____**

   Weight   Reps   Weight   Reps   Weight   Reps

1.   X   1.   X   1.   X
2.   X   2.   X   2.   X
3.   X   3.   X   3.   X
4.   X   4.   X   4.   X
5.   X   5.   X   5.   X

Aerobic Workout   **ABS**

Exercise   Time   Exercise_____

1._____   ____Min/Hr Set/Reps 1.____   2.____   3.____

2._____   ____Min/Hr Exercise_____

                             Set/Reps 1.____   2.____   3.____

Saturday_____   Month____ Yr___

Exercise_____   **Exercise_____**   **Exercise_____**

   Weight   Reps   Weight   Reps   Weight   Reps

1.   X   1.   X   1.   X
2.   X   2.   X   2.   X
3.   X   3.   X   3.   X
4.   X   4.   X   4.   X
5.   X   5.   X   5.   X

Exercise_____   **Exercise_____**   **Exercise_____**

   Weight   Reps   Weight   Reps   Weight   Reps

1.   X   1.   X   1.   X
2.   X   2.   X   2.   X
3.   X   3.   X   3.   X
4.   X   4.   X   4.   X
5.   X   5.   X   5.   X

Exercise_____   **Exercise_____**   **Exercise_____**

   Weight   Reps   Weight   Reps   Weight   Reps

1.   X   1.   X   1.   X
2.   X   2.   X   2.   X
3.   X   3.   X   3.   X
4.   X   4.   X   4.   X
5.   X   5.   X   5.   X

Exercise_____   **Exercise_____**   **Exercise_____**

   Weight   Reps   Weight   Reps   Weight   Reps

1.   X   1.   X   1.   X
2.   X   2.   X   2.   X
3.   X   3.   X   3.   X
4.   X   4.   X   4.   X
5.   X   5.   X   5.   X

Aerobic Workout   **ABS**

Exercise   Time   Exercise_____

1._____   ____Min/Hr Set/Reps 1._____   2._____   3._____

2._____   ____Min/Hr Exercise_____

                            Set/Reps 1._____   2._____   3._____

Notes

Sunday_____   **Month_____ Yr___**

Exercise_____   **Exercise_____**   **Exercise_____**

   Weight   Reps   Weight   Reps   Weight   Reps

1.   X   1.   X   1.   X
2.   X   2.   X   2.   X
3.   X   3.   X   3.   X
4.   X   4.   X   4.   X
5.   X   5.   X   5.   X

Exercise_____   **Exercise_____**   **Exercise_____**

   Weight   Reps   Weight   Reps   Weight   Reps

1.   X   1.   X   1.   X
2.   X   2.   X   2.   X
3.   X   3.   X   3.   X
4.   X   4.   X   4.   X
5.   X   5.   X   5.   X

Exercise_____   **Exercise_____**   **Exercise_____**

   Weight   Reps   Weight   Reps   Weight   Reps

1.   X   1.   X   1.   X
2.   X   2.   X   2.   X
3.   X   3.   X   3.   X
4.   X   4.   X   4.   X
5.   X   5.   X   5.   X

Exercise_____   **Exercise_____**   **Exercise_____**

   Weight   Reps   Weight   Reps   Weight   Reps

1.   X   1.   X   1.   X
2.   X   2.   X   2.   X
3.   X   3.   X   3.   X
4.   X   4.   X   4.   X
5.   X   5.   X   5.   X

Aerobic Workout   **ABS**

Exercise   Time   Exercise_____

1._____   ____Min/Hr   Set/Reps 1.____   2.____   3.____

2._____   ____Min/Hr   Exercise_____

                               Set/Reps 1.____   2.____   3.____

Monday_____   Month_____ Yr___

Exercise_____   **Exercise_____**   **Exercise_____**

  Weight   Reps   Weight   Reps   Weight   Reps

1.	X	1.	X	1.	X
2.	X	2.	X	2.	X
3.	X	3.	X	3.	X
4.	X	4.	X	4.	X
5.	X	5.	X	5.	X

Exercise_____   **Exercise_____**   **Exercise_____**

  Weight   Reps   Weight   Reps   Weight   Reps

1.	X	1.	X	1.	X
2.	X	2.	X	2.	X
3.	X	3.	X	3.	X
4.	X	4.	X	4.	X
5.	X	5.	X	5.	X

Exercise_____   **Exercise_____**   **Exercise_____**

  Weight   Reps   Weight   Reps   Weight   Reps

1.	X	1.	X	1.	X
2.	X	2.	X	2.	X
3.	X	3.	X	3.	X
4.	X	4.	X	4.	X
5.	X	5.	X	5.	X

Exercise_____   **Exercise_____**   **Exercise_____**

  Weight   Reps   Weight   Reps   Weight   Reps

1.	X	1.	X	1.	X
2.	X	2.	X	2.	X
3.	X	3.	X	3.	X
4.	X	4.	X	4.	X
5.	X	5.	X	5.	X

Aerobic Workout   **ABS**

Exercise   Time   Exercise_____

1._____   ____Min/Hr   Set/Reps   1.____   2.____   3.____

2._____   ____Min/Hr   Exercise_____

                                 Set/Reps   1.____   2.____   3.____

Tuesday_____   Month_____ Yr___

Exercise_____   **Exercise**_____   **Exercise**_____

   Weight   Reps   Weight   Reps   Weight   Reps

1.	X	1.	X	1.	X
2.	X	2.	X	2.	X
3.	X	3.	X	3.	X
4.	X	4.	X	4.	X
5.	X	5.	X	5.	X

Exercise_____   **Exercise**_____   **Exercise**_____

   Weight   Reps   Weight   Reps   Weight   Reps

1.	X	1.	X	1.	X
2.	X	2.	X	2.	X
3.	X	3.	X	3.	X
4.	X	4.	X	4.	X
5.	X	5.	X	5.	X

Exercise_____   **Exercise**_____   **Exercise**_____

   Weight   Reps   Weight   Reps   Weight   Reps

1.	X	1.	X	1.	X
2.	X	2.	X	2.	X
3.	X	3.	X	3.	X
4.	X	4.	X	4.	X
5.	X	5.	X	5.	X

Exercise_____   **Exercise**_____   **Exercise**_____

   Weight   Reps   Weight   Reps   Weight   Reps

1.	X	1.	X	1.	X
2.	X	2.	X	2.	X
3.	X	3.	X	3.	X
4.	X	4.	X	4.	X
5.	X	5.	X	5.	X

Aerobic Workout   **ABS**

Exercise   Time   Exercise_____

1._____ ____Min/Hr Set/Reps 1.____ 2.____   3.____

2._____ ____Min/Hr Exercise_____

                      Set/Reps 1.____ 2.____   3.____

Wednesday_____   Month_____ Yr___

Exercise_____   **Exercise_____**   **Exercise_____**

   Weight   Reps   Weight   Reps   Weight   Reps

1.   X   1.   X   1.   X
2.   X   2.   X   2.   X
3.   X   3.   X   3.   X
4.   X   4.   X   4.   X
5.   X   5.   X   5.   X

Exercise_____   **Exercise_____**   **Exercise_____**

   Weight   Reps   Weight   Reps   Weight   Reps

1.   X   1.   X   1.   X
2.   X   2.   X   2.   X
3.   X   3.   X   3.   X
4.   X   4.   X   4.   X
5.   X   5.   X   5.   X

Exercise_____   **Exercise_____**   **Exercise_____**

   Weight   Reps   Weight   Reps   Weight   Reps

1.   X   1.   X   1.   X
2.   X   2.   X   2.   X
3.   X   3.   X   3.   X
4.   X   4.   X   4.   X
5.   X   5.   X   5.   X

Exercise_____   **Exercise_____**   **Exercise_____**

   Weight   Reps   Weight   Reps   Weight   Reps

1.   X   1.   X   1.   X
2.   X   2.   X   2.   X
3.   X   3.   X   3.   X
4.   X   4.   X   4.   X
5.   X   5.   X   5.   X

Aerobic Workout   **ABS**

Exercise   Time   Exercise_____

1._____   ____Min/Hr Set/Reps 1.____   2.____   3.____

2._____   ____Min/Hr Exercise_____

                                 Set/Reps 1.____   2.____   3.____

Thursday_____   Month_____ Yr___

Exercise_____   **Exercise_____**   **Exercise_____**

   Weight   Reps   Weight   Reps   Weight   Reps

1.   X   1.   X   1.   X
2.   X   2.   X   2.   X
3.   X   3.   X   3.   X
4.   X   4.   X   4.   X
5.   X   5.   X   5.   X

Exercise_____   **Exercise_____**   **Exercise_____**

   Weight   Reps   Weight   Reps   Weight   Reps

1.   X   1.   X   1.   X
2.   X   2.   X   2.   X
3.   X   3.   X   3.   X
4.   X   4.   X   4.   X
5.   X   5.   X   5.   X

Exercise_____   **Exercise_____**   **Exercise_____**

   Weight   Reps   Weight   Reps   Weight   Reps

1.   X   1.   X   1.   X
2.   X   2.   X   2.   X
3.   X   3.   X   3.   X
4.   X   4.   X   4.   X
5.   X   5.   X   5.   X

Exercise_____   **Exercise_____**   **Exercise_____**

   Weight   Reps   Weight   Reps   Weight   Reps

1.   X   1.   X   1.   X
2.   X   2.   X   2.   X
3.   X   3.   X   3.   X
4.   X   4.   X   4.   X
5.   X   5.   X   5.   X

Aerobic Workout   **ABS**

Exercise   Time   Exercise_____

1._____   ____Min/Hr Set/Reps 1.____   2.____   3.____

2._____   ____Min/Hr Exercise_____

                           Set/Reps 1.____   2.____   3.____

Friday_____   Month____ Yr___

Exercise_____   **Exercise**_____   **Exercise**_____

   Weight   Reps   Weight   Reps   Weight   Reps

1.   X   1.   X   1.   X
2.   X   2.   X   2.   X
3.   X   3.   X   3.   X
4.   X   4.   X   4.   X
5.   X   5.   X   5.   X

Exercise_____   **Exercise**_____   **Exercise**_____

   Weight   Reps   Weight   Reps   Weight   Reps

1.   X   1.   X   1.   X
2.   X   2.   X   2.   X
3.   X   3.   X   3.   X
4.   X   4.   X   4.   X
5.   X   5.   X   5.   X

Exercise_____   **Exercise**_____   **Exercise**_____

   Weight   Reps   Weight   Reps   Weight   Reps

1.   X   1.   X   1.   X
2.   X   2.   X   2.   X
3.   X   3.   X   3.   X
4.   X   4.   X   4.   X
5.   X   5.   X   5.   X

Exercise_____   **Exercise**_____   **Exercise**_____

   Weight   Reps   Weight   Reps   Weight   Reps

1.   X   1.   X   1.   X
2.   X   2.   X   2.   X
3.   X   3.   X   3.   X
4.   X   4.   X   4.   X
5.   X   5.   X   5.   X

Aerobic Workout   **ABS**

Exercise   Time   Exercise_____

1._____   ____Min/Hr   Set/Reps   1._____   2._____   3._____

2._____   ____Min/Hr   Exercise_____

                                 Set/Reps   1._____   2._____   3._____

23

Saturday_____   Month____ Yr___

Exercise_____   **Exercise_____**   **Exercise_____**

   Weight   Reps   Weight   Reps   Weight   Reps

1.   X   1.   X   1.   X
2.   X   2.   X   2.   X
3.   X   3.   X   3.   X
4.   X   4.   X   4.   X
5.   X   5.   X   5.   X

Exercise_____   **Exercise_____**   **Exercise_____**

   Weight   Reps   Weight   Reps   Weight   Reps

1.   X   1.   X   1.   X
2.   X   2.   X   2.   X
3.   X   3.   X   3.   X
4.   X   4.   X   4.   X
5.   X   5.   X   5.   X

Exercise_____   **Exercise_____**   **Exercise_____**

   Weight   Reps   Weight   Reps   Weight   Reps

1.   X   1.   X   1.   X
2.   X   2.   X   2.   X
3.   X   3.   X   3.   X
4.   X   4.   X   4.   X
5.   X   5.   X   5.   X

Exercise_____   **Exercise_____**   **Exercise_____**

   Weight   Reps   Weight   Reps   Weight   Reps

1.   X   1.   X   1.   X
2.   X   2.   X   2.   X
3.   X   3.   X   3.   X
4.   X   4.   X   4.   X
5.   X   5.   X   5.   X

Aerobic Workout   **ABS**

Exercise   Time   Exercise_____

1._____   ____Min/Hr Set/Reps 1.____   2.____   3.____

2._____   ____Min/Hr Exercise_____

                              Set/Reps 1.____   2.____   3.____

Notes

_____

_____

_____

_____

_____

_____

_____

_____

_____

_____

_____

_____

_____

_____

_____

_____

_____

Sunday_____   Month_____ Yr___

Exercise_____   **Exercise_____**   **Exercise_____**

   Weight   Reps   Weight   Reps   Weight   Reps

1.   X   1.   X   1.   X
2.   X   2.   X   2.   X
3.   X   3.   X   3.   X
4.   X   4.   X   4.   X
5.   X   5.   X   5.   X

Exercise_____   **Exercise_____**   **Exercise_____**

   Weight   Reps   Weight   Reps   Weight   Reps

1.   X   1.   X   1.   X
2.   X   2.   X   2.   X
3.   X   3.   X   3.   X
4.   X   4.   X   4.   X
5.   X   5.   X   5.   X

Exercise_____   **Exercise_____**   **Exercise_____**

   Weight   Reps   Weight   Reps   Weight   Reps

1.   X   1.   X   1.   X
2.   X   2.   X   2.   X
3.   X   3.   X   3.   X
4.   X   4.   X   4.   X
5.   X   5.   X   5.   X

Exercise_____   **Exercise_____**   **Exercise_____**

   Weight   Reps   Weight   Reps   Weight   Reps

1.   X   1.   X   1.   X
2.   X   2.   X   2.   X
3.   X   3.   X   3.   X
4.   X   4.   X   4.   X
5.   X   5.   X   5.   X

Aerobic Workout   **ABS**

Exercise   Time   Exercise_____

1._____   ____Min/Hr Set/Reps 1.____ 2.____   3.____

2._____   ____Min/Hr Exercise_____

                            Set/Reps 1.____ 2.____   3.____

Monday_____   Month_____ Yr___

Exercise_____   **Exercise_____**   **Exercise_____**

   Weight   Reps   Weight   Reps   Weight   Reps

1.   X   1.   X   1.   X
2.   X   2.   X   2.   X
3.   X   3.   X   3.   X
4.   X   4.   X   4.   X
5.   X   5.   X   5.   X

Exercise_____   **Exercise_____**   **Exercise_____**

   Weight   Reps   Weight   Reps   Weight   Reps

1.   X   1.   X   1.   X
2.   X   2.   X   2.   X
3.   X   3.   X   3.   X
4.   X   4.   X   4.   X
5.   X   5.   X   5.   X

Exercise_____   **Exercise_____**   **Exercise_____**

   Weight   Reps   Weight   Reps   Weight   Reps

1.   X   1.   X   1.   X
2.   X   2.   X   2.   X
3.   X   3.   X   3.   X
4.   X   4.   X   4.   X
5.   X   5.   X   5.   X

Exercise_____   **Exercise_____**   **Exercise_____**

   Weight   Reps   Weight   Reps   Weight   Reps

1.   X   1.   X   1.   X
2.   X   2.   X   2.   X
3.   X   3.   X   3.   X
4.   X   4.   X   4.   X
5.   X   5.   X   5.   X

Aerobic Workout   **ABS**

Exercise   Time   Exercise_____

1._____   ____Min/Hr   Set/Reps 1.____   2.____   3.____

2._____   ____Min/Hr   Exercise_____

                              Set/Reps 1.____   2.____   3.____

27

Tuesday_____   Month_____ Yr___

Exercise_____   **Exercise_____**   **Exercise_____**

   Weight   Reps   Weight   Reps   Weight   Reps

1.   X   1.   X   1.   X
2.   X   2.   X   2.   X
3.   X   3.   X   3.   X
4.   X   4.   X   4.   X
5.   X   5.   X   5.   X

Exercise_____   **Exercise_____**   **Exercise_____**

   Weight   Reps   Weight   Reps   Weight   Reps

1.   X   1.   X   1.   X
2.   X   2.   X   2.   X
3.   X   3.   X   3.   X
4.   X   4.   X   4.   X
5.   X   5.   X   5.   X

Exercise_____   **Exercise_____**   **Exercise_____**

   Weight   Reps   Weight   Reps   Weight   Reps

1.   X   1.   X   1.   X
2.   X   2.   X   2.   X
3.   X   3.   X   3.   X
4.   X   4.   X   4.   X
5.   X   5.   X   5.   X

Exercise_____   **Exercise_____**   **Exercise_____**

   Weight   Reps   Weight   Reps   Weight   Reps

1.   X   1.   X   1.   X
2.   X   2.   X   2.   X
3.   X   3.   X   3.   X
4.   X   4.   X   4.   X
5.   X   5.   X   5.   X

Aerobic Workout   **ABS**

Exercise   Time   Exercise_____

1._____   ____Min/Hr   Set/Reps   1.____   2.____   3.____

2._____   ____Min/Hr   Exercise_____

                              Set/Reps   1.____   2.____   3.____

Wednesday_____   Month____Yr___

Exercise_____   **Exercise_____**   **Exercise_____**

    Weight   Reps   Weight   Reps   Weight   Reps

1.   X   1.   X   1.   X
2.   X   2.   X   2.   X
3.   X   3.   X   3.   X
4.   X   4.   X   4.   X
5.   X   5.   X   5.   X

Exercise_____   **Exercise_____**   **Exercise_____**

    Weight   Reps   Weight   Reps   Weight   Reps

1.   X   1.   X   1.   X
2.   X   2.   X   2.   X
3.   X   3.   X   3.   X
4.   X   4.   X   4.   X
5.   X   5.   X   5.   X

Exercise_____   **Exercise_____**   **Exercise_____**

    Weight   Reps   Weight   Reps   Weight   Reps

1.   X   1.   X   1.   X
2.   X   2.   X   2.   X
3.   X   3.   X   3.   X
4.   X   4.   X   4.   X
5.   X   5.   X   5.   X

Exercise_____   **Exercise_____**   **Exercise_____**

    Weight   Reps   Weight   Reps   Weight   Reps

1.   X   1.   X   1.   X
2.   X   2.   X   2.   X
3.   X   3.   X   3.   X
4.   X   4.   X   4.   X
5.   X   5.   X   5.   X

Aerobic Workout   **ABS**

Exercise   Time   Exercise_____

1._____   ____Min/Hr Set/Reps 1.____   2.____   3.____

2._____   ____Min/Hr Exercise_____

                             Set/Reps 1.____   2.____   3.____

Thursday_____   Month_____ Yr___

Exercise_____   **Exercise_____**   **Exercise_____**

   Weight   Reps   Weight   Reps   Weight   Reps

1.   X   1.   X   1.   X
2.   X   2.   X   2.   X
3.   X   3.   X   3.   X
4.   X   4.   X   4.   X
5.   X   5.   X   5.   X

Exercise_____   **Exercise_____**   **Exercise_____**

   Weight   Reps   Weight   Reps   Weight   Reps

1.   X   1.   X   1.   X
2.   X   2.   X   2.   X
3.   X   3.   X   3.   X
4.   X   4.   X   4.   X
5.   X   5.   X   5.   X

Exercise_____   **Exercise_____**   **Exercise_____**

   Weight   Reps   Weight   Reps   Weight   Reps

1.   X   1.   X   1.   X
2.   X   2.   X   2.   X
3.   X   3.   X   3.   X
4.   X   4.   X   4.   X
5.   X   5.   X   5.   X

Exercise_____   **Exercise_____**   **Exercise_____**

   Weight   Reps   Weight   Reps   Weight   Reps

1.   X   1.   X   1.   X
2.   X   2.   X   2.   X
3.   X   3.   X   3.   X
4.   X   4.   X   4.   X
5.   X   5.   X   5.   X

Aerobic Workout   **ABS**

Exercise   Time   Exercise_____

1._____   ____Min/Hr Set/Reps 1.____   2.____   3.____

2._____   ____Min/Hr Exercise_____

                           Set/Reps 1.____   2.____   3.____

Friday_____   Month_____ Yr___

Exercise_____   **Exercise_____**   **Exercise_____**

   Weight   Reps   Weight   Reps   Weight   Reps

1.	X		1.	X		1.	X
2.	X		2.	X		2.	X
3.	X		3.	X		3.	X
4.	X		4.	X		4.	X
5.	X		5.	X		5.	X

Exercise_____   **Exercise_____**   **Exercise_____**

   Weight   Reps   Weight   Reps   Weight   Reps

1.	X		1.	X		1.	X
2.	X		2.	X		2.	X
3.	X		3.	X		3.	X
4.	X		4.	X		4.	X
5.	X		5.	X		5.	X

Exercise_____   **Exercise_____**   **Exercise_____**

   Weight   Reps   Weight   Reps   Weight   Reps

1.	X		1.	X		1.	X
2.	X		2.	X		2.	X
3.	X		3.	X		3.	X
4.	X		4.	X		4.	X
5.	X		5.	X		5.	X

Exercise_____   **Exercise_____**   **Exercise_____**

   Weight   Reps   Weight   Reps   Weight   Reps

1.	X		1.	X		1.	X
2.	X		2.	X		2.	X
3.	X		3.	X		3.	X
4.	X		4.	X		4.	X
5.	X		5.	X		5.	X

Aerobic Workout   **ABS**

Exercise   Time   Exercise_____

1._____ ____Min/Hr Set/Reps 1.____ 2.____   3.____

2._____ ____Min/Hr Exercise_____

                       Set/Reps 1.____ 2.____   3.____

Saturday_____   Month_____ Yr___

Exercise_____   **Exercise_____**   **Exercise_____**

   Weight   Reps   Weight   Reps   Weight   Reps

1.   X   1.   X   1.   X
2.   X   2.   X   2.   X
3.   X   3.   X   3.   X
4.   X   4.   X   4.   X
5.   X   5.   X   5.   X

Exercise_____   **Exercise_____**   **Exercise_____**

   Weight   Reps   Weight   Reps   Weight   Reps

1.   X   1.   X   1.   X
2.   X   2.   X   2.   X
3.   X   3.   X   3.   X
4.   X   4.   X   4.   X
5.   X   5.   X   5.   X

Exercise_____   **Exercise_____**   **Exercise_____**

   Weight   Reps   Weight   Reps   Weight   Reps

1.   X   1.   X   1.   X
2.   X   2.   X   2.   X
3.   X   3.   X   3.   X
4.   X   4.   X   4.   X
5.   X   5.   X   5.   X

Exercise_____   **Exercise_____**   **Exercise_____**

   Weight   Reps   Weight   Reps   Weight   Reps

1.   X   1.   X   1.   X
2.   X   2.   X   2.   X
3.   X   3.   X   3.   X
4.   X   4.   X   4.   X
5.   X   5.   X   5.   X

Aerobic Workout   **ABS**

Exercise   Time   Exercise_____

1._____   ____Min/Hr Set/Reps 1.____   2.____   3.____

2._____   ____Min/Hr Exercise_____

                           Set/Reps 1.____   2.____   3.____

Notes

_____

_____

_____

_____

_____

_____

_____

_____

_____

_____

_____

_____

_____

_____

_____

_____

_____

_____

_____

Sunday_____   Month____   Yr___

Exercise_____   **Exercise_____**   **Exercise_____**

  Weight   Reps   Weight   Reps   Weight   Reps

1.   X   1.   X   1.   X
2.   X   2.   X   2.   X
3.   X   3.   X   3.   X
4.   X   4.   X   4.   X
5.   X   5.   X   5.   X

Exercise_____   **Exercise_____**   **Exercise_____**

  Weight   Reps   Weight   Reps   Weight   Reps

1.   X   1.   X   1.   X
2.   X   2.   X   2.   X
3.   X   3.   X   3.   X
4.   X   4.   X   4.   X
5.   X   5.   X   5.   X

Exercise_____   **Exercise_____**   **Exercise_____**

  Weight   Reps   Weight   Reps   Weight   Reps

1.   X   1.   X   1.   X
2.   X   2.   X   2.   X
3.   X   3.   X   3.   X
4.   X   4.   X   4.   X
5.   X   5.   X   5.   X

Exercise_____   **Exercise_____**   **Exercise_____**

  Weight   Reps   Weight   Reps   Weight   Reps

1.   X   1.   X   1.   X
2.   X   2.   X   2.   X
3.   X   3.   X   3.   X
4.   X   4.   X   4.   X
5.   X   5.   X   5.   X

Aerobic Workout   **ABS**

Exercise   Time   Exercise_____

1._____   ____Min/Hr   Set/Reps   1.____   2.____   3.____

2._____   ____Min/Hr   Exercise_____

                        Set/Reps   1.____   2.____   3.____

Monday_____   Month____ Yr___

Exercise_____   **Exercise**_____   **Exercise**_____

   Weight   Reps   Weight   Reps   Weight   Reps

1.   X   1.   X   1.   X
2.   X   2.   X   2.   X
3.   X   3.   X   3.   X
4.   X   4.   X   4.   X
5.   X   5.   X   5.   X

Exercise_____   **Exercise**_____   **Exercise**_____

   Weight   Reps   Weight   Reps   Weight   Reps

1.   X   1.   X   1.   X
2.   X   2.   X   2.   X
3.   X   3.   X   3.   X
4.   X   4.   X   4.   X
5.   X   5.   X   5.   X

Exercise_____   **Exercise**_____   **Exercise**_____

   Weight   Reps   Weight   Reps   Weight   Reps

1.   X   1.   X   1.   X
2.   X   2.   X   2.   X
3.   X   3.   X   3.   X
4.   X   4.   X   4.   X
5.   X   5.   X   5.   X

Exercise_____   **Exercise**_____   **Exercise**_____

   Weight   Reps   Weight   Reps   Weight   Reps

1.   X   1.   X   1.   X
2.   X   2.   X   2.   X
3.   X   3.   X   3.   X
4.   X   4.   X   4.   X
5.   X   5.   X   5.   X

Aerobic Workout   **ABS**

Exercise   Time   Exercise_____

1._____   ____Min/Hr Set/Reps 1.____   2.____   3.____

2._____   ____Min/Hr Exercise_____

                                 Set/Reps 1.____   2.____   3.____

Tuesday_____   Month____ Yr___

Exercise_____   **Exercise_____**   **Exercise_____**

   Weight   Reps   Weight   Reps   Weight   Reps

1.   X   1.   X   1.   X
2.   X   2.   X   2.   X
3.   X   3.   X   3.   X
4.   X   4.   X   4.   X
5.   X   5.   X   5.   X

Exercise_____   **Exercise_____**   **Exercise_____**

   Weight   Reps   Weight   Reps   Weight   Reps

1.   X   1.   X   1.   X
2.   X   2.   X   2.   X
3.   X   3.   X   3.   X
4.   X   4.   X   4.   X
5.   X   5.   X   5.   X

Exercise_____   **Exercise_____**   **Exercise_____**

   Weight   Reps   Weight   Reps   Weight   Reps

1.   X   1.   X   1.   X
2.   X   2.   X   2.   X
3.   X   3.   X   3.   X
4.   X   4.   X   4.   X
5.   X   5.   X   5.   X

Exercise_____   **Exercise_____**   **Exercise_____**

   Weight   Reps   Weight   Reps   Weight   Reps

1.   X   1.   X   1.   X
2.   X   2.   X   2.   X
3.   X   3.   X   3.   X
4.   X   4.   X   4.   X
5.   X   5.   X   5.   X

Aerobic Workout   **ABS**

Exercise   Time   Exercise_____

1._____   ____Min/Hr   Set/Reps   1.____   2.____   3.____

2._____   ____Min/Hr   Exercise_____

                              Set/Reps   1.____   2.____   3.____

Wednesday_____   Month_____ Yr___

Exercise_____   **Exercise_____**   **Exercise_____**

  Weight   Reps   Weight   Reps   Weight   Reps

1.	X	1.	X	1.	X
2.	X	2.	X	2.	X
3.	X	3.	X	3.	X
4.	X	4.	X	4.	X
5.	X	5.	X	5.	X

Exercise_____   **Exercise_____**   **Exercise_____**

  Weight   Reps   Weight   Reps   Weight   Reps

1.	X	1.	X	1.	X
2.	X	2.	X	2.	X
3.	X	3.	X	3.	X
4.	X	4.	X	4.	X
5.	X	5.	X	5.	X

Exercise_____   **Exercise_____**   **Exercise_____**

  Weight   Reps   Weight   Reps   Weight   Reps

1.	X	1.	X	1.	X
2.	X	2.	X	2.	X
3.	X	3.	X	3.	X
4.	X	4.	X	4.	X
5.	X	5.	X	5.	X

Exercise_____   **Exercise_____**   **Exercise_____**

  Weight   Reps   Weight   Reps   Weight   Reps

1.	X	1.	X	1.	X
2.	X	2.	X	2.	X
3.	X	3.	X	3.	X
4.	X	4.	X	4.	X
5.	X	5.	X	5.	X

Aerobic Workout   **ABS**

Exercise   Time   Exercise_____

1._____ ____Min/Hr Set/Reps 1.____ 2.____   3.____

2._____ ____Min/Hr Exercise_____

                       Set/Reps 1.____ 2.____   3.____

Thursday_____   Month_____ Yr___

Exercise_____   **Exercise_____**   **Exercise_____**

   Weight   Reps   Weight   Reps   Weight   Reps

1.   X   1.   X   1.   X
2.   X   2.   X   2.   X
3.   X   3.   X   3.   X
4.   X   4.   X   4.   X
5.   X   5.   X   5.   X

Exercise_____   **Exercise_____**   **Exercise_____**

   Weight   Reps   Weight   Reps   Weight   Reps

1.   X   1.   X   1.   X
2.   X   2.   X   2.   X
3.   X   3.   X   3.   X
4.   X   4.   X   4.   X
5.   X   5.   X   5.   X

Exercise_____   **Exercise_____**   **Exercise_____**

   Weight   Reps   Weight   Reps   Weight   Reps

1.   X   1.   X   1.   X
2.   X   2.   X   2.   X
3.   X   3.   X   3.   X
4.   X   4.   X   4.   X
5.   X   5.   X   5.   X

Exercise_____   **Exercise_____**   **Exercise_____**

   Weight   Reps   Weight   Reps   Weight   Reps

1.   X   1.   X   1.   X
2.   X   2.   X   2.   X
3.   X   3.   X   3.   X
4.   X   4.   X   4.   X
5.   X   5.   X   5.   X

Aerobic Workout   **ABS**

Exercise   Time   Exercise_____

1._____   ____Min/Hr Set/Reps 1.____ 2.____   3.____

2._____   ____Min/Hr Exercise_____

                              Set/Reps 1.____ 2.____   3.____

Friday_____   Month_____ Yr___

Exercise_____   **Exercise_____**   **Exercise_____**

    Weight   Reps   Weight   Reps   Weight   Reps

1.   X   1.   X   1.   X
2.   X   2.   X   2.   X
3.   X   3.   X   3.   X
4.   X   4.   X   4.   X
5.   X   5.   X   5.   X

Exercise_____   **Exercise_____**   **Exercise_____**

    Weight   Reps   Weight   Reps   Weight   Reps

1.   X   1.   X   1.   X
2.   X   2.   X   2.   X
3.   X   3.   X   3.   X
4.   X   4.   X   4.   X
5.   X   5.   X   5.   X

Exercise_____   **Exercise_____**   **Exercise_____**

    Weight   Reps   Weight   Reps   Weight   Reps

1.   X   1.   X   1.   X
2.   X   2.   X   2.   X
3.   X   3.   X   3.   X
4.   X   4.   X   4.   X
5.   X   5.   X   5.   X

Exercise_____   **Exercise_____**   **Exercise_____**

    Weight   Reps   Weight   Reps   Weight   Reps

1.   X   1.   X   1.   X
2.   X   2.   X   2.   X
3.   X   3.   X   3.   X
4.   X   4.   X   4.   X
5.   X   5.   X   5.   X

Aerobic Workout   **ABS**

Exercise   Time   Exercise_____

1._____   ____Min/Hr Set/Reps 1.____   2.____   3.____

2._____   ____Min/Hr Exercise_____

                              Set/Reps 1.____   2.____   3.____

Saturday_____   Month_____ Yr___

Exercise_____   **Exercise_____**   **Exercise_____**

  Weight   Reps   Weight   Reps   Weight   Reps

1.	X		1.	X		1.	X	
2.	X		2.	X		2.	X	
3.	X		3.	X		3.	X	
4.	X		4.	X		4.	X	
5.	X		5.	X		5.	X	

Exercise_____   **Exercise_____**   **Exercise_____**

  Weight   Reps   Weight   Reps   Weight   Reps

1.	X		1.	X		1.	X	
2.	X		2.	X		2.	X	
3.	X		3.	X		3.	X	
4.	X		4.	X		4.	X	
5.	X		5.	X		5.	X	

Exercise_____   **Exercise_____**   **Exercise_____**

  Weight   Reps   Weight   Reps   Weight   Reps

1.	X		1.	X		1.	X	
2.	X		2.	X		2.	X	
3.	X		3.	X		3.	X	
4.	X		4.	X		4.	X	
5.	X		5.	X		5.	X	

Exercise_____   **Exercise_____**   **Exercise_____**

  Weight   Reps   Weight   Reps   Weight   Reps

1.	X		1.	X		1.	X	
2.	X		2.	X		2.	X	
3.	X		3.	X		3.	X	
4.	X		4.	X		4.	X	
5.	X		5.	X		5.	X	

Aerobic Workout   **ABS**

Exercise   Time   Exercise_____

1._____   ____Min/Hr   Set/Reps   1.____   2.____   3.____

2._____   ____Min/Hr   Exercise_____

                                          Set/Reps   1.____   2.____   3.____

40

Notes

_____

_____

_____

_____

_____

_____

_____

_____

_____

_____

_____

_____

_____

_____

_____

_____

_____

Sunday_____   Month____ Yr___

Exercise_____   **Exercise_____**   **Exercise_____**

Weight	Reps	Weight	Reps	Weight	Reps
1. X		1. X		1. X	
2. X		2. X		2. X	
3. X		3. X		3. X	
4. X		4. X		4. X	
5. X		5. X		5. X	

Exercise_____   **Exercise_____**   **Exercise_____**

Weight	Reps	Weight	Reps	Weight	Reps
1. X		1. X		1. X	
2. X		2. X		2. X	
3. X		3. X		3. X	
4. X		4. X		4. X	
5. X		5. X		5. X	

Exercise_____   **Exercise_____**   **Exercise_____**

Weight	Reps	Weight	Reps	Weight	Reps
1. X		1. X		1. X	
2. X		2. X		2. X	
3. X		3. X		3. X	
4. X		4. X		4. X	
5. X		5. X		5. X	

Exercise_____   **Exercise_____**   **Exercise_____**

Weight	Reps	Weight	Reps	Weight	Reps
1. X		1. X		1. X	
2. X		2. X		2. X	
3. X		3. X		3. X	
4. X		4. X		4. X	
5. X		5. X		5. X	

Aerobic Workout   **ABS**

Exercise	Time	Exercise_____

1._____   ____Min/Hr   Set/Reps   1.____   2.____   3.____

Exercise_____

2._____   ____Min/Hr

Set/Reps   1.____   2.____   3.____

Monday_____   Month_____ Yr___

Exercise_____   **Exercise_____**   **Exercise_____**

  Weight   Reps   Weight   Reps   Weight   Reps

1.   X   1.   X   1.   X
2.   X   2.   X   2.   X
3.   X   3.   X   3.   X
4.   X   4.   X   4.   X
5.   X   5.   X   5.   X

Exercise_____   **Exercise_____**   **Exercise_____**

  Weight   Reps   Weight   Reps   Weight   Reps

1.   X   1.   X   1.   X
2.   X   2.   X   2.   X
3.   X   3.   X   3.   X
4.   X   4.   X   4.   X
5.   X   5.   X   5.   X

Exercise_____   **Exercise_____**   **Exercise_____**

  Weight   Reps   Weight   Reps   Weight   Reps

1.   X   1.   X   1.   X
2.   X   2.   X   2.   X
3.   X   3.   X   3.   X
4.   X   4.   X   4.   X
5.   X   5.   X   5.   X

Exercise_____   **Exercise_____**   **Exercise_____**

  Weight   Reps   Weight   Reps   Weight   Reps

1.   X   1.   X   1.   X
2.   X   2.   X   2.   X
3.   X   3.   X   3.   X
4.   X   4.   X   4.   X
5.   X   5.   X   5.   X

Aerobic Workout   **ABS**

Exercise   Time   Exercise_____

1._____   ____Min/Hr   Set/Reps   1.____   2.____   3.____

2._____   ____Min/Hr   Exercise_____

                             Set/Reps   1.____   2.____   3.____

Tuesday_____   Month_____ Yr___

Exercise_____ **Exercise**_____ **Exercise**_____

   Weight   Reps   Weight   Reps   Weight   Reps

1.   X   1.   X   1.   X
2.   X   2.   X   2.   X
3.   X   3.   X   3.   X
4.   X   4.   X   4.   X
5.   X   5.   X   5.   X

Exercise_____ **Exercise**_____ **Exercise**_____

   Weight   Reps   Weight   Reps   Weight   Reps

1.   X   1.   X   1.   X
2.   X   2.   X   2.   X
3.   X   3.   X   3.   X
4.   X   4.   X   4.   X
5.   X   5.   X   5.   X

Exercise_____ **Exercise**_____ **Exercise**_____

   Weight   Reps   Weight   Reps   Weight   Reps

1.   X   1.   X   1.   X
2.   X   2.   X   2.   X
3.   X   3.   X   3.   X
4.   X   4.   X   4.   X
5.   X   5.   X   5.   X

Exercise_____ **Exercise**_____ **Exercise**_____

   Weight   Reps   Weight   Reps   Weight   Reps

1.   X   1.   X   1.   X
2.   X   2.   X   2.   X
3.   X   3.   X   3.   X
4.   X   4.   X   4.   X
5.   X   5.   X   5.   X

Aerobic Workout   **ABS**

Exercise   Time   Exercise_____

1._____ ____Min/Hr Set/Reps 1.____ 2.____   3.____

2._____ ____Min/Hr Exercise_____

                            Set/Reps 1.____ 2.____   3.____

Wednesday_____   Month_____ Yr___

Exercise_____   **Exercise_____**   **Exercise_____**

   Weight   Reps   Weight   Reps   Weight   Reps

1.   X   1.   X   1.   X
2.   X   2.   X   2.   X
3.   X   3.   X   3.   X
4.   X   4.   X   4.   X
5.   X   5.   X   5.   X

Exercise_____   **Exercise_____**   **Exercise_____**

   Weight   Reps   Weight   Reps   Weight   Reps

1.   X   1.   X   1.   X
2.   X   2.   X   2.   X
3.   X   3.   X   3.   X
4.   X   4.   X   4.   X
5.   X   5.   X   5.   X

Exercise_____   **Exercise_____**   **Exercise_____**

   Weight   Reps   Weight   Reps   Weight   Reps

1.   X   1.   X   1.   X
2.   X   2.   X   2.   X
3.   X   3.   X   3.   X
4.   X   4.   X   4.   X
5.   X   5.   X   5.   X

Exercise_____   **Exercise_____**   **Exercise_____**

   Weight   Reps   Weight   Reps   Weight   Reps

1.   X   1.   X   1.   X
2.   X   2.   X   2.   X
3.   X   3.   X   3.   X
4.   X   4.   X   4.   X
5.   X   5.   X   5.   X

Aerobic Workout   **ABS**

Exercise   Time   Exercise_____

1._____   ____Min/Hr Set/Reps 1.____   2.____   3.____

2._____   ____Min/Hr Exercise_____

                          Set/Reps 1.____   2.____   3.____

Thursday_____   Month_____ Yr___

Exercise_____   **Exercise**_____   **Exercise**_____

   Weight   Reps   Weight   Reps   Weight   Reps

1.   X   1.   X   1.   X
2.   X   2.   X   2.   X
3.   X   3.   X   3.   X
4.   X   4.   X   4.   X
5.   X   5.   X   5.   X

Exercise_____   **Exercise**_____   **Exercise**_____

   Weight   Reps   Weight   Reps   Weight   Reps

1.   X   1.   X   1.   X
2.   X   2.   X   2.   X
3.   X   3.   X   3.   X
4.   X   4.   X   4.   X
5.   X   5.   X   5.   X

Exercise_____   **Exercise**_____   **Exercise**_____

   Weight   Reps   Weight   Reps   Weight   Reps

1.   X   1.   X   1.   X
2.   X   2.   X   2.   X
3.   X   3.   X   3.   X
4.   X   4.   X   4.   X
5.   X   5.   X   5.   X

Exercise_____   **Exercise**_____   **Exercise**_____

   Weight   Reps   Weight   Reps   Weight   Reps

1.   X   1.   X   1.   X
2.   X   2.   X   2.   X
3.   X   3.   X   3.   X
4.   X   4.   X   4.   X
5.   X   5.   X   5.   X

Aerobic Workout   **ABS**

Exercise   Time   Exercise_____

1._____ ____Min/Hr Set/Reps 1.____   2.____   3.____

2._____ ____Min/Hr Exercise_____

                            Set/Reps 1.____   2.____   3.____

Friday_____   Month_____ Yr___

Exercise_____   **Exercise_____**   **Exercise_____**

   Weight   Reps   Weight   Reps   Weight   Reps

1.	X	1.	X	1.	X
2.	X	2.	X	2.	X
3.	X	3.	X	3.	X
4.	X	4.	X	4.	X
5.	X	5.	X	5.	X

Exercise_____   **Exercise_____**   **Exercise_____**

   Weight   Reps   Weight   Reps   Weight   Reps

1.	X	1.	X	1.	X
2.	X	2.	X	2.	X
3.	X	3.	X	3.	X
4.	X	4.	X	4.	X
5.	X	5.	X	5.	X

Exercise_____   **Exercise_____**   **Exercise_____**

   Weight   Reps   Weight   Reps   Weight   Reps

1.	X	1.	X	1.	X
2.	X	2.	X	2.	X
3.	X	3.	X	3.	X
4.	X	4.	X	4.	X
5.	X	5.	X	5.	X

Exercise_____   **Exercise_____**   **Exercise_____**

   Weight   Reps   Weight   Reps   Weight   Reps

1.	X	1.	X	1.	X
2.	X	2.	X	2.	X
3.	X	3.	X	3.	X
4.	X	4.	X	4.	X
5.	X	5.	X	5.	X

Aerobic Workout   **ABS**

Exercise   Time   Exercise_____

1._____   ____Min/Hr Set/Reps 1.____   2.____   3.____

2._____   ____Min/Hr Exercise_____

                              Set/Reps 1.____   2.____   3.____

Saturday_____   Month____ Yr___

Exercise_____   **Exercise_____**   **Exercise_____**

   Weight   Reps   Weight   Reps   Weight   Reps

1.   X   1.   X   1.   X
2.   X   2.   X   2.   X
3.   X   3.   X   3.   X
4.   X   4.   X   4.   X
5.   X   5.   X   5.   X

Exercise_____   **Exercise_____**   **Exercise_____**

   Weight   Reps   Weight   Reps   Weight   Reps

1.   X   1.   X   1.   X
2.   X   2.   X   2.   X
3.   X   3.   X   3.   X
4.   X   4.   X   4.   X
5.   X   5.   X   5.   X

Exercise_____   **Exercise_____**   **Exercise_____**

   Weight   Reps   Weight   Reps   Weight   Reps

1.   X   1.   X   1.   X
2.   X   2.   X   2.   X
3.   X   3.   X   3.   X
4.   X   4.   X   4.   X
5.   X   5.   X   5.   X

Exercise_____   **Exercise_____**   **Exercise_____**

   Weight   Reps   Weight   Reps   Weight   Reps

1.   X   1.   X   1.   X
2.   X   2.   X   2.   X
3.   X   3.   X   3.   X
4.   X   4.   X   4.   X
5.   X   5.   X   5.   X

Aerobic Workout   **ABS**

Exercise   Time   Exercise_____

1._____   ____Min/Hr Set/Reps 1.____   2.____   3.____

2._____   ____Min/Hr Exercise_____

                              Set/Reps 1.____   2.____   3.____

Notes

_____

_____

_____

_____

_____

_____

_____

_____

_____

_____

_____

_____

_____

_____

_____

_____

_____

Sunday_____   Month_____ Yr___

Exercise_____ **Exercise**_____ **Exercise**_____

   Weight   Reps   Weight   Reps   Weight   Reps

1.   X   1.   X   1.   X
2.   X   2.   X   2.   X
3.   X   3.   X   3.   X
4.   X   4.   X   4.   X
5.   X   5.   X   5.   X

Exercise_____ **Exercise**_____ **Exercise**_____

   Weight   Reps   Weight   Reps   Weight   Reps

1.   X   1.   X   1.   X
2.   X   2.   X   2.   X
3.   X   3.   X   3.   X
4.   X   4.   X   4.   X
5.   X   5.   X   5.   X

Exercise_____ **Exercise**_____ **Exercise**_____

   Weight   Reps   Weight   Reps   Weight   Reps

1.   X   1.   X   1.   X
2.   X   2.   X   2.   X
3.   X   3.   X   3.   X
4.   X   4.   X   4.   X
5.   X   5.   X   5.   X

Exercise_____ **Exercise**_____ **Exercise**_____

   Weight   Reps   Weight   Reps   Weight   Reps

1.   X   1.   X   1.   X
2.   X   2.   X   2.   X
3.   X   3.   X   3.   X
4.   X   4.   X   4.   X
5.   X   5.   X   5.   X

Aerobic Workout   **ABS**

Exercise   Time   Exercise_____

1._____ ____Min/Hr Set/Reps 1.____   2.____   3.____

2._____ ____Min/Hr Exercise_____

                             Set/Reps 1.____   2.____   3.____

Monday_____   Month____ Yr___

Exercise_____   **Exercise_____**   **Exercise_____**

   Weight   Reps   Weight   Reps   Weight   Reps

1.   X   1.   X   1.   X
2.   X   2.   X   2.   X
3.   X   3.   X   3.   X
4.   X   4.   X   4.   X
5.   X   5.   X   5.   X

Exercise_____   **Exercise_____**   **Exercise_____**

   Weight   Reps   Weight   Reps   Weight   Reps

1.   X   1.   X   1.   X
2.   X   2.   X   2.   X
3.   X   3.   X   3.   X
4.   X   4.   X   4.   X
5.   X   5.   X   5.   X

Exercise_____   **Exercise_____**   **Exercise_____**

   Weight   Reps   Weight   Reps   Weight   Reps

1.   X   1.   X   1.   X
2.   X   2.   X   2.   X
3.   X   3.   X   3.   X
4.   X   4.   X   4.   X
5.   X   5.   X   5.   X

Exercise_____   **Exercise_____**   **Exercise_____**

   Weight   Reps   Weight   Reps   Weight   Reps

1.   X   1.   X   1.   X
2.   X   2.   X   2.   X
3.   X   3.   X   3.   X
4.   X   4.   X   4.   X
5.   X   5.   X   5.   X

Aerobic Workout   **ABS**

Exercise   Time   Exercise_____

1._____   ____Min/Hr   Set/Reps   1.____   2.____   3.____

2._____   ____Min/Hr   Exercise_____

                              Set/Reps   1.____   2.____   3.____

51

Tuesday_____   Month_____ Yr___

Exercise_____ **Exercise**_____ **Exercise**_____

   Weight   Reps   Weight   Reps   Weight   Reps

1.   X   1.   X   1.   X
2.   X   2.   X   2.   X
3.   X   3.   X   3.   X
4.   X   4.   X   4.   X
5.   X   5.   X   5.   X

Exercise_____ **Exercise**_____ **Exercise**_____

   Weight   Reps   Weight   Reps   Weight   Reps

1.   X   1.   X   1.   X
2.   X   2.   X   2.   X
3.   X   3.   X   3.   X
4.   X   4.   X   4.   X
5.   X   5.   X   5.   X

Exercise_____ **Exercise**_____ **Exercise**_____

   Weight   Reps   Weight   Reps   Weight   Reps

1.   X   1.   X   1.   X
2.   X   2.   X   2.   X
3.   X   3.   X   3.   X
4.   X   4.   X   4.   X
5.   X   5.   X   5.   X

Exercise_____ **Exercise**_____ **Exercise**_____

   Weight   Reps   Weight   Reps   Weight   Reps

1.   X   1.   X   1.   X
2.   X   2.   X   2.   X
3.   X   3.   X   3.   X
4.   X   4.   X   4.   X
5.   X   5.   X   5.   X

Aerobic Workout   **ABS**

Exercise   Time   Exercise_____

1._____   ____Min/Hr   Set/Reps   1.____   2.____   3.____

2._____   ____Min/Hr   Exercise_____

                              Set/Reps   1.____   2.____   3.____

Wednesday_____   Month_____ Yr___

Exercise_____   **Exercise_____**   **Exercise_____**

   Weight   Reps   Weight   Reps   Weight   Reps

1.	X	1.	X	1.	X
2.	X	2.	X	2.	X
3.	X	3.	X	3.	X
4.	X	4.	X	4.	X
5.	X	5.	X	5.	X

Exercise_____   **Exercise_____**   **Exercise_____**

   Weight   Reps   Weight   Reps   Weight   Reps

1.	X	1.	X	1.	X
2.	X	2.	X	2.	X
3.	X	3.	X	3.	X
4.	X	4.	X	4.	X
5.	X	5.	X	5.	X

Exercise_____   **Exercise_____**   **Exercise_____**

   Weight   Reps   Weight   Reps   Weight   Reps

1.	X	1.	X	1.	X
2.	X	2.	X	2.	X
3.	X	3.	X	3.	X
4.	X	4.	X	4.	X
5.	X	5.	X	5.	X

Exercise_____   **Exercise_____**   **Exercise_____**

   Weight   Reps   Weight   Reps   Weight   Reps

1.	X	1.	X	1.	X
2.	X	2.	X	2.	X
3.	X	3.	X	3.	X
4.	X	4.	X	4.	X
5.	X	5.	X	5.	X

Aerobic Workout   **ABS**

Exercise   Time   Exercise_____

1._____   _____Min/Hr   Set/Reps 1._____   2._____   3._____

2._____   _____Min/Hr   Exercise_____

                                 Set/Reps 1._____   2._____   3._____

Thursday_____   Month_____ Yr___

Exercise_____   **Exercise_____**   **Exercise_____**

   Weight   Reps   Weight   Reps   Weight   Reps

1.	X	1.	X	1.	X
2.	X	2.	X	2.	X
3.	X	3.	X	3.	X
4.	X	4.	X	4.	X
5.	X	5.	X	5.	X

Exercise_____   **Exercise_____**   **Exercise_____**

   Weight   Reps   Weight   Reps   Weight   Reps

1.	X	1.	X	1.	X
2.	X	2.	X	2.	X
3.	X	3.	X	3.	X
4.	X	4.	X	4.	X
5.	X	5.	X	5.	X

Exercise_____   **Exercise_____**   **Exercise_____**

   Weight   Reps   Weight   Reps   Weight   Reps

1.	X	1.	X	1.	X
2.	X	2.	X	2.	X
3.	X	3.	X	3.	X
4.	X	4.	X	4.	X
5.	X	5.	X	5.	X

Exercise_____   **Exercise_____**   **Exercise_____**

   Weight   Reps   Weight   Reps   Weight   Reps

1.	X	1.	X	1.	X
2.	X	2.	X	2.	X
3.	X	3.	X	3.	X
4.	X	4.	X	4.	X
5.	X	5.	X	5.	X

Aerobic Workout   **ABS**

Exercise   Time   Exercise_____

1._____   ____Min/Hr   Set/Reps 1.____   2.____   3.____

2._____   ____Min/Hr   Exercise_____

                                      Set/Reps 1.____   2.____   3.____

Friday_____   Month_____ Yr___

Exercise_____   **Exercise_____**   **Exercise_____**

   Weight   Reps   Weight   Reps   Weight   Reps

1.   X   1.   X   1.   X
2.   X   2.   X   2.   X
3.   X   3.   X   3.   X
4.   X   4.   X   4.   X
5.   X   5.   X   5.   X

Exercise_____   **Exercise_____**   **Exercise_____**

   Weight   Reps   Weight   Reps   Weight   Reps

1.   X   1.   X   1.   X
2.   X   2.   X   2.   X
3.   X   3.   X   3.   X
4.   X   4.   X   4.   X
5.   X   5.   X   5.   X

Exercise_____   **Exercise_____**   **Exercise_____**

   Weight   Reps   Weight   Reps   Weight   Reps

1.   X   1.   X   1.   X
2.   X   2.   X   2.   X
3.   X   3.   X   3.   X
4.   X   4.   X   4.   X
5.   X   5.   X   5.   X

Exercise_____   **Exercise_____**   **Exercise_____**

   Weight   Reps   Weight   Reps   Weight   Reps

1.   X   1.   X   1.   X
2.   X   2.   X   2.   X
3.   X   3.   X   3.   X
4.   X   4.   X   4.   X
5.   X   5.   X   5.   X

Aerobic Workout   **ABS**

Exercise   Time   Exercise_____

1._____ ____Min/Hr Set/Reps 1.____ 2.____ 3.____

2._____ ____Min/Hr Exercise_____

                       Set/Reps 1.____ 2.____ 3.____

Saturday_____   Month_____ Yr___

Exercise_____   **Exercise_____**   **Exercise_____**

   Weight   Reps   Weight   Reps   Weight   Reps

1.   X   1.   X   1.   X
2.   X   2.   X   2.   X
3.   X   3.   X   3.   X
4.   X   4.   X   4.   X
5.   X   5.   X   5.   X

Exercise_____   **Exercise_____**   **Exercise_____**

   Weight   Reps   Weight   Reps   Weight   Reps

1.   X   1.   X   1.   X
2.   X   2.   X   2.   X
3.   X   3.   X   3.   X
4.   X   4.   X   4.   X
5.   X   5.   X   5.   X

Exercise_____   **Exercise_____**   **Exercise_____**

   Weight   Reps   Weight   Reps   Weight   Reps

1.   X   1.   X   1.   X
2.   X   2.   X   2.   X
3.   X   3.   X   3.   X
4.   X   4.   X   4.   X
5.   X   5.   X   5.   X

Exercise_____   **Exercise_____**   **Exercise_____**

   Weight   Reps   Weight   Reps   Weight   Reps

1.   X   1.   X   1.   X
2.   X   2.   X   2.   X
3.   X   3.   X   3.   X
4.   X   4.   X   4.   X
5.   X   5.   X   5.   X

Aerobic Workout   **ABS**

Exercise   Time   Exercise_____

1._____   ____Min/Hr   Set/Reps 1.____   2.____   3.____

2._____   ____Min/Hr   Exercise_____

                           Set/Reps 1.____   2.____   3.____

56

Notes

_____

_____

_____

_____

_____

_____

_____

_____

_____

_____

_____

_____

_____

_____

_____

_____

_____

Sunday_____   Month_____ Yr___

Exercise_____   **Exercise_____**   **Exercise_____**

   Weight   Reps   Weight   Reps   Weight   Reps

1.   X   1.   X   1.   X
2.   X   2.   X   2.   X
3.   X   3.   X   3.   X
4.   X   4.   X   4.   X
5.   X   5.   X   5.   X

Exercise_____   **Exercise_____**   **Exercise_____**

   Weight   Reps   Weight   Reps   Weight   Reps

1.   X   1.   X   1.   X
2.   X   2.   X   2.   X
3.   X   3.   X   3.   X
4.   X   4.   X   4.   X
5.   X   5.   X   5.   X

Exercise_____   **Exercise_____**   **Exercise_____**

   Weight   Reps   Weight   Reps   Weight   Reps

1.   X   1.   X   1.   X
2.   X   2.   X   2.   X
3.   X   3.   X   3.   X
4.   X   4.   X   4.   X
5.   X   5.   X   5.   X

Exercise_____   **Exercise_____**   **Exercise_____**

   Weight   Reps   Weight   Reps   Weight   Reps

1.   X   1.   X   1.   X
2.   X   2.   X   2.   X
3.   X   3.   X   3.   X
4.   X   4.   X   4.   X
5.   X   5.   X   5.   X

Aerobic Workout   **ABS**

Exercise   Time   Exercise_____

1._____   ____Min/Hr Set/Reps 1.____   2.____   3.____

2._____   ____Min/Hr Exercise_____

                             Set/Reps 1.____   2.____   3.____

Monday_____   Month_____ Yr___

Exercise_____   **Exercise_____**   **Exercise_____**

   Weight   Reps   Weight   Reps   Weight   Reps

1.   X   1.   X   1.   X
2.   X   2.   X   2.   X
3.   X   3.   X   3.   X
4.   X   4.   X   4.   X
5.   X   5.   X   5.   X

Exercise_____   **Exercise_____**   **Exercise_____**

   Weight   Reps   Weight   Reps   Weight   Reps

1.   X   1.   X   1.   X
2.   X   2.   X   2.   X
3.   X   3.   X   3.   X
4.   X   4.   X   4.   X
5.   X   5.   X   5.   X

Exercise_____   **Exercise_____**   **Exercise_____**

   Weight   Reps   Weight   Reps   Weight   Reps

1.   X   1.   X   1.   X
2.   X   2.   X   2.   X
3.   X   3.   X   3.   X
4.   X   4.   X   4.   X
5.   X   5.   X   5.   X

Exercise_____   **Exercise_____**   **Exercise_____**

   Weight   Reps   Weight   Reps   Weight   Reps

1.   X   1.   X   1.   X
2.   X   2.   X   2.   X
3.   X   3.   X   3.   X
4.   X   4.   X   4.   X
5.   X   5.   X   5.   X

Aerobic Workout   **ABS**

Exercise   Time   Exercise_____

1._____ ____Min/Hr Set/Reps 1.____ 2.____   3.____

2._____ ____Min/Hr Exercise_____

                        Set/Reps 1.____ 2.____   3.____

Tuesday_____   Month____ Yr___

Exercise_____   **Exercise**_____   **Exercise**_____

   Weight   Reps   Weight   Reps   Weight   Reps

1.   X   1.   X   1.   X
2.   X   2.   X   2.   X
3.   X   3.   X   3.   X
4.   X   4.   X   4.   X
5.   X   5.   X   5.   X

Exercise_____   **Exercise**_____   **Exercise**_____

   Weight   Reps   Weight   Reps   Weight   Reps

1.   X   1.   X   1.   X
2.   X   2.   X   2.   X
3.   X   3.   X   3.   X
4.   X   4.   X   4.   X
5.   X   5.   X   5.   X

Exercise_____   **Exercise**_____   **Exercise**_____

   Weight   Reps   Weight   Reps   Weight   Reps

1.   X   1.   X   1.   X
2.   X   2.   X   2.   X
3.   X   3.   X   3.   X
4.   X   4.   X   4.   X
5.   X   5.   X   5.   X

Exercise_____   **Exercise**_____   **Exercise**_____

   Weight   Reps   Weight   Reps   Weight   Reps

1.   X   1.   X   1.   X
2.   X   2.   X   2.   X
3.   X   3.   X   3.   X
4.   X   4.   X   4.   X
5.   X   5.   X   5.   X

Aerobic Workout   **ABS**

Exercise   Time   Exercise_____

1._____   ____Min/Hr   Set/Reps 1.____   2.____   3.____

2._____   ____Min/Hr   Exercise_____

                            Set/Reps 1.____   2.____   3.____

60

Wednesday_____   Month____ Yr___

Exercise_____   **Exercise_____**   **Exercise_____**

  Weight   Reps   Weight   Reps   Weight   Reps

1.   X   1.   X   1.   X
2.   X   2.   X   2.   X
3.   X   3.   X   3.   X
4.   X   4.   X   4.   X
5.   X   5.   X   5.   X

Exercise_____   **Exercise_____**   **Exercise_____**

  Weight   Reps   Weight   Reps   Weight   Reps

1.   X   1.   X   1.   X
2.   X   2.   X   2.   X
3.   X   3.   X   3.   X
4.   X   4.   X   4.   X
5.   X   5.   X   5.   X

Exercise_____   **Exercise_____**   **Exercise_____**

  Weight   Reps   Weight   Reps   Weight   Reps

1.   X   1.   X   1.   X
2.   X   2.   X   2.   X
3.   X   3.   X   3.   X
4.   X   4.   X   4.   X
5.   X   5.   X   5.   X

Exercise_____   **Exercise_____**   **Exercise_____**

  Weight   Reps   Weight   Reps   Weight   Reps

1.   X   1.   X   1.   X
2.   X   2.   X   2.   X
3.   X   3.   X   3.   X
4.   X   4.   X   4.   X
5.   X   5.   X   5.   X

Aerobic Workout   **ABS**

Exercise   Time   Exercise_____

1._____   ____Min/Hr   Set/Reps 1.____   2.____   3.____

2._____   ____Min/Hr   Exercise_____

                              Set/Reps 1.____   2.____   3.____

Thursday_____   Month_____ Yr___

Exercise_____   **Exercise**_____   **Exercise**_____

   Weight   Reps   Weight   Reps   Weight   Reps

1.   X   1.   X   1.   X
2.   X   2.   X   2.   X
3.   X   3.   X   3.   X
4.   X   4.   X   4.   X
5.   X   5.   X   5.   X

Exercise_____   **Exercise**_____   **Exercise**_____

   Weight   Reps   Weight   Reps   Weight   Reps

1.   X   1.   X   1.   X
2.   X   2.   X   2.   X
3.   X   3.   X   3.   X
4.   X   4.   X   4.   X
5.   X   5.   X   5.   X

Exercise_____   **Exercise**_____   **Exercise**_____

   Weight   Reps   Weight   Reps   Weight   Reps

1.   X   1.   X   1.   X
2.   X   2.   X   2.   X
3.   X   3.   X   3.   X
4.   X   4.   X   4.   X
5.   X   5.   X   5.   X

Exercise_____   **Exercise**_____   **Exercise**_____

   Weight   Reps   Weight   Reps   Weight   Reps

1.   X   1.   X   1.   X
2.   X   2.   X   2.   X
3.   X   3.   X   3.   X
4.   X   4.   X   4.   X
5.   X   5.   X   5.   X

Aerobic Workout   **ABS**

Exercise   Time   Exercise_____

1._____   ____Min/Hr   Set/Reps 1.____   2.____   3.____

2._____   ____Min/Hr   Exercise_____

                                 Set/Reps 1.____   2.____   3.____

Friday_____   Month_____ Yr___

Exercise_____   **Exercise**_____   **Exercise**_____

   Weight   Reps   Weight   Reps   Weight   Reps

1.	X	1.	X	1.	X
2.	X	2.	X	2.	X
3.	X	3.	X	3.	X
4.	X	4.	X	4.	X
5.	X	5.	X	5.	X

Exercise_____   **Exercise**_____   **Exercise**_____

   Weight   Reps   Weight   Reps   Weight   Reps

1.	X	1.	X	1.	X
2.	X	2.	X	2.	X
3.	X	3.	X	3.	X
4.	X	4.	X	4.	X
5.	X	5.	X	5.	X

Exercise_____   **Exercise**_____   **Exercise**_____

   Weight   Reps   Weight   Reps   Weight   Reps

1.	X	1.	X	1.	X
2.	X	2.	X	2.	X
3.	X	3.	X	3.	X
4.	X	4.	X	4.	X
5.	X	5.	X	5.	X

Exercise_____   **Exercise**_____   **Exercise**_____

   Weight   Reps   Weight   Reps   Weight   Reps

1.	X	1.	X	1.	X
2.	X	2.	X	2.	X
3.	X	3.	X	3.	X
4.	X	4.	X	4.	X
5.	X	5.	X	5.	X

Aerobic Workout   **ABS**

Exercise   Time   Exercise_____

1._____   ____Min/Hr Set/Reps 1.____   2.____   3.____

2._____   ____Min/Hr Exercise_____

                              Set/Reps 1.____   2.____   3.____

Saturday_____   Month_____ Yr___

Exercise_____   **Exercise**_____   **Exercise**_____

   Weight   Reps   Weight   Reps   Weight   Reps

1.	X	1.	X	1.	X
2.	X	2.	X	2.	X
3.	X	3.	X	3.	X
4.	X	4.	X	4.	X
5.	X	5.	X	5.	X

Exercise_____   **Exercise**_____   **Exercise**_____

   Weight   Reps   Weight   Reps   Weight   Reps

1.	X	1.	X	1.	X
2.	X	2.	X	2.	X
3.	X	3.	X	3.	X
4.	X	4.	X	4.	X
5.	X	5.	X	5.	X

Exercise_____   **Exercise**_____   **Exercise**_____

   Weight   Reps   Weight   Reps   Weight   Reps

1.	X	1.	X	1.	X
2.	X	2.	X	2.	X
3.	X	3.	X	3.	X
4.	X	4.	X	4.	X
5.	X	5.	X	5.	X

Exercise_____   **Exercise**_____   **Exercise**_____

   Weight   Reps   Weight   Reps   Weight   Reps

1.	X	1.	X	1.	X
2.	X	2.	X	2.	X
3.	X	3.	X	3.	X
4.	X	4.	X	4.	X
5.	X	5.	X	5.	X

Aerobic Workout   **ABS**

Exercise   Time   Exercise_____

1._____   ____Min/Hr   Set/Reps   1._____   2._____   3._____

2._____   ____Min/Hr   Exercise_____

                                  Set/Reps   1._____   2._____   3._____

Notes

_____

_____

_____

_____

_____

_____

_____

_____

_____

_____

_____

_____

_____

_____

_____

_____

_____

_____

Sunday_____   Month_____ Yr___

Exercise_____   **Exercise_____**   **Exercise_____**

   Weight   Reps   Weight   Reps   Weight   Reps

1.   X   1.   X   1.   X
2.   X   2.   X   2.   X
3.   X   3.   X   3.   X
4.   X   4.   X   4.   X
5.   X   5.   X   5.   X

Exercise_____   **Exercise_____**   **Exercise_____**

   Weight   Reps   Weight   Reps   Weight   Reps

1.   X   1.   X   1.   X
2.   X   2.   X   2.   X
3.   X   3.   X   3.   X
4.   X   4.   X   4.   X
5.   X   5.   X   5.   X

Exercise_____   **Exercise_____**   **Exercise_____**

   Weight   Reps   Weight   Reps   Weight   Reps

1.   X   1.   X   1.   X
2.   X   2.   X   2.   X
3.   X   3.   X   3.   X
4.   X   4.   X   4.   X
5.   X   5.   X   5.   X

Exercise_____   **Exercise_____**   **Exercise_____**

   Weight   Reps   Weight   Reps   Weight   Reps

1.   X   1.   X   1.   X
2.   X   2.   X   2.   X
3.   X   3.   X   3.   X
4.   X   4.   X   4.   X
5.   X   5.   X   5.   X

Aerobic Workout   **ABS**

Exercise   Time   Exercise_____

1._____   ____Min/Hr Set/Reps 1.____   2.____   3.____

2._____   ____Min/Hr Exercise_____

                                  Set/Reps 1.____   2.____   3.____

Monday_____   Month_____ Yr___

Exercise_____ **Exercise_____** **Exercise_____**

	Weight	Reps		Weight	Reps		Weight	Reps
1.	X		1.	X		1.	X	
2.	X		2.	X		2.	X	
3.	X		3.	X		3.	X	
4.	X		4.	X		4.	X	
5.	X		5.	X		5.	X	

Exercise_____ **Exercise_____** **Exercise_____**

	Weight	Reps		Weight	Reps		Weight	Reps
1.	X		1.	X		1.	X	
2.	X		2.	X		2.	X	
3.	X		3.	X		3.	X	
4.	X		4.	X		4.	X	
5.	X		5.	X		5.	X	

Exercise_____ **Exercise_____** **Exercise_____**

	Weight	Reps		Weight	Reps		Weight	Reps
1.	X		1.	X		1.	X	
2.	X		2.	X		2.	X	
3.	X		3.	X		3.	X	
4.	X		4.	X		4.	X	
5.	X		5.	X		5.	X	

Exercise_____ **Exercise_____** **Exercise_____**

	Weight	Reps		Weight	Reps		Weight	Reps
1.	X		1.	X		1.	X	
2.	X		2.	X		2.	X	
3.	X		3.	X		3.	X	
4.	X		4.	X		4.	X	
5.	X		5.	X		5.	X	

Aerobic Workout   **ABS**

Exercise   Time   Exercise_____

1._____   ____Min/Hr Set/Reps 1._____   2._____   3._____

2._____   ____Min/Hr Exercise_____

                                Set/Reps 1._____   2._____   3._____

67

Tuesday_____   Month_____ Yr___

Exercise_____   **Exercise_____**   **Exercise_____**

   Weight   Reps   Weight   Reps   Weight Reps

1.   X   1.   X   1.   X
2.   X   2.   X   2.   X
3.   X   3.   X   3.   X
4.   X   4.   X   4.   X
5.   X   5.   X   5.   X

Exercise_____   **Exercise_____**   **Exercise_____**

   Weight   Reps   Weight   Reps   Weight Reps

1.   X   1.   X   1.   X
2.   X   2.   X   2.   X
3.   X   3.   X   3.   X
4.   X   4.   X   4.   X
5.   X   5.   X   5.   X

Exercise_____   **Exercise_____**   **Exercise_____**

   Weight   Reps   Weight   Reps   Weight Reps

1.   X   1.   X   1.   X
2.   X   2.   X   2.   X
3.   X   3.   X   3.   X
4.   X   4.   X   4.   X
5.   X   5.   X   5.   X

Exercise_____   **Exercise_____**   **Exercise_____**

   Weight   Reps   Weight   Reps   Weight Reps

1.   X   1.   X   1.   X
2.   X   2.   X   2.   X
3.   X   3.   X   3.   X
4.   X   4.   X   4.   X
5.   X   5.   X   5.   X

Aerobic Workout   **ABS**

Exercise   Time   Exercise_____

1._____   ____Min/Hr Set/Reps 1.____   2.____   3.____

2._____   ____Min/Hr Exercise_____

                          Set/Reps 1.____   2.____   3.____

Wednesday_____   Month_____ Yr___

Exercise_____   **Exercise_____**   **Exercise_____**

   Weight   Reps   Weight   Reps   Weight   Reps

1.   X   1.   X   1.   X
2.   X   2.   X   2.   X
3.   X   3.   X   3.   X
4.   X   4.   X   4.   X
5.   X   5.   X   5.   X

Exercise_____   **Exercise_____**   **Exercise_____**

   Weight   Reps   Weight   Reps   Weight   Reps

1.   X   1.   X   1.   X
2.   X   2.   X   2.   X
3.   X   3.   X   3.   X
4.   X   4.   X   4.   X
5.   X   5.   X   5.   X

Exercise_____   **Exercise_____**   **Exercise_____**

   Weight   Reps   Weight   Reps   Weight   Reps

1.   X   1.   X   1.   X
2.   X   2.   X   2.   X
3.   X   3.   X   3.   X
4.   X   4.   X   4.   X
5.   X   5.   X   5.   X

Exercise_____   **Exercise_____**   **Exercise_____**

   Weight   Reps   Weight   Reps   Weight   Reps

1.   X   1.   X   1.   X
2.   X   2.   X   2.   X
3.   X   3.   X   3.   X
4.   X   4.   X   4.   X
5.   X   5.   X   5.   X

Aerobic Workout   **ABS**

Exercise   Time   Exercise_____

1._____   ____Min/Hr Set/Reps 1._____   2._____   3._____

2._____   ____Min/Hr Exercise_____

                                Set/Reps 1._____   2._____   3._____

Thursday_____   Month_____ Yr___

Exercise_____   **Exercise_____**   **Exercise_____**

   Weight   Reps   Weight   Reps   Weight   Reps

1.   X   1.   X   1.   X
2.   X   2.   X   2.   X
3.   X   3.   X   3.   X
4.   X   4.   X   4.   X
5.   X   5.   X   5.   X

Exercise_____   **Exercise_____**   **Exercise_____**

   Weight   Reps   Weight   Reps   Weight   Reps

1.   X   1.   X   1.   X
2.   X   2.   X   2.   X
3.   X   3.   X   3.   X
4.   X   4.   X   4.   X
5.   X   5.   X   5.   X

Exercise_____   **Exercise_____**   **Exercise_____**

   Weight   Reps   Weight   Reps   Weight   Reps

1.   X   1.   X   1.   X
2.   X   2.   X   2.   X
3.   X   3.   X   3.   X
4.   X   4.   X   4.   X
5.   X   5.   X   5.   X

Exercise_____   **Exercise_____**   **Exercise_____**

   Weight   Reps   Weight   Reps   Weight   Reps

1.   X   1.   X   1.   X
2.   X   2.   X   2.   X
3.   X   3.   X   3.   X
4.   X   4.   X   4.   X
5.   X   5.   X   5.   X

Aerobic Workout   **ABS**

Exercise   Time   Exercise_____

1._____ ____Min/Hr   Set/Reps 1.____ 2.____   3.____

2._____ ____Min/Hr   Exercise_____

                             Set/Reps 1.____ 2.____   3.____

Friday_____   Month_____ Yr___

Exercise_____   **Exercise_____**   **Exercise_____**

   Weight   Reps   Weight   Reps   Weight   Reps

1.	X	1.	X	1.	X
2.	X	2.	X	2.	X
3.	X	3.	X	3.	X
4.	X	4.	X	4.	X
5.	X	5.	X	5.	X

Exercise_____   **Exercise_____**   **Exercise_____**

   Weight   Reps   Weight   Reps   Weight   Reps

1.	X	1.	X	1.	X
2.	X	2.	X	2.	X
3.	X	3.	X	3.	X
4.	X	4.	X	4.	X
5.	X	5.	X	5.	X

Exercise_____   **Exercise_____**   **Exercise_____**

   Weight   Reps   Weight   Reps   Weight   Reps

1.	X	1.	X	1.	X
2.	X	2.	X	2.	X
3.	X	3.	X	3.	X
4.	X	4.	X	4.	X
5.	X	5.	X	5.	X

Exercise_____   **Exercise_____**   **Exercise_____**

   Weight   Reps   Weight   Reps   Weight   Reps

1.	X	1.	X	1.	X
2.	X	2.	X	2.	X
3.	X	3.	X	3.	X
4.	X	4.	X	4.	X
5.	X	5.	X	5.	X

Aerobic Workout   **ABS**

Exercise   Time   Exercise_____

1._____ ____Min/Hr Set/Reps 1.____ 2.____ 3.____

2._____ ____Min/Hr Exercise_____

                          Set/Reps 1.____ 2.____ 3.____

Saturday_____   Month_____ Yr___

Exercise_____   **Exercise**_____   **Exercise**_____

  Weight   Reps   Weight   Reps   Weight   Reps

1.   X   1.   X   1.   X
2.   X   2.   X   2.   X
3.   X   3.   X   3.   X
4.   X   4.   X   4.   X
5.   X   5.   X   5.   X

Exercise_____   **Exercise**_____   **Exercise**_____

  Weight   Reps   Weight   Reps   Weight   Reps

1.   X   1.   X   1.   X
2.   X   2.   X   2.   X
3.   X   3.   X   3.   X
4.   X   4.   X   4.   X
5.   X   5.   X   5.   X

Exercise_____   **Exercise**_____   **Exercise**_____

  Weight   Reps   Weight   Reps   Weight   Reps

1.   X   1.   X   1.   X
2.   X   2.   X   2.   X
3.   X   3.   X   3.   X
4.   X   4.   X   4.   X
5.   X   5.   X   5.   X

Exercise_____   **Exercise**_____   **Exercise**_____

  Weight   Reps   Weight   Reps   Weight   Reps

1.   X   1.   X   1.   X
2.   X   2.   X   2.   X
3.   X   3.   X   3.   X
4.   X   4.   X   4.   X
5.   X   5.   X   5.   X

Aerobic Workout   **ABS**

Exercise   Time   Exercise_____

1._____   ____Min/Hr Set/Reps 1.____   2.____   3.____

2._____   ____Min/Hr Exercise_____

                           Set/Reps 1.____   2.____   3.____

Notes

_____

_____

_____

_____

_____

_____

_____

_____

_____

_____

_____

_____

_____

_____

_____

_____

_____

Sunday_____   Month_____ Yr___

Exercise_____   **Exercise_____**   **Exercise_____**

   Weight   Reps   Weight   Reps   Weight   Reps

1.   X   1.   X   1.   X
2.   X   2.   X   2.   X
3.   X   3.   X   3.   X
4.   X   4.   X   4.   X
5.   X   5.   X   5.   X

Exercise_____   **Exercise_____**   **Exercise_____**

   Weight   Reps   Weight   Reps   Weight   Reps

1.   X   1.   X   1.   X
2.   X   2.   X   2.   X
3.   X   3.   X   3.   X
4.   X   4.   X   4.   X
5.   X   5.   X   5.   X

Exercise_____   **Exercise_____**   **Exercise_____**

   Weight   Reps   Weight   Reps   Weight   Reps

1.   X   1.   X   1.   X
2.   X   2.   X   2.   X
3.   X   3.   X   3.   X
4.   X   4.   X   4.   X
5.   X   5.   X   5.   X

Exercise_____   **Exercise_____**   **Exercise_____**

   Weight   Reps   Weight   Reps   Weight   Reps

1.   X   1.   X   1.   X
2.   X   2.   X   2.   X
3.   X   3.   X   3.   X
4.   X   4.   X   4.   X
5.   X   5.   X   5.   X

Aerobic Workout   **ABS**

Exercise   Time   Exercise_____

1._____   ____Min/Hr Set/Reps 1.____   2.____   3.____

2._____   ____Min/Hr Exercise_____

                           Set/Reps 1.____   2.____   3.____

Monday_____   Month_____ Yr___

Exercise_____   Exercise_____   Exercise_____

	Weight	Reps		Weight	Reps		Weight	Reps
1.	X		1.	X		1.	X	
2.	X		2.	X		2.	X	
3.	X		3.	X		3.	X	
4.	X		4.	X		4.	X	
5.	X		5.	X		5.	X	

Exercise_____   Exercise_____   Exercise_____

	Weight	Reps		Weight	Reps		Weight	Reps
1.	X		1.	X		1.	X	
2.	X		2.	X		2.	X	
3.	X		3.	X		3.	X	
4.	X		4.	X		4.	X	
5.	X		5.	X		5.	X	

Exercise_____   Exercise_____   Exercise_____

	Weight	Reps		Weight	Reps		Weight	Reps
1.	X		1.	X		1.	X	
2.	X		2.	X		2.	X	
3.	X		3.	X		3.	X	
4.	X		4.	X		4.	X	
5.	X		5.	X		5.	X	

Exercise_____   Exercise_____   Exercise_____

	Weight	Reps		Weight	Reps		Weight	Reps
1.	X		1.	X		1.	X	
2.	X		2.	X		2.	X	
3.	X		3.	X		3.	X	
4.	X		4.	X		4.	X	
5.	X		5.	X		5.	X	

Aerobic Workout   **ABS**

Exercise   Time   Exercise_____

1._____   ____Min/Hr   Set/Reps   1.____   2.____   3.____

2._____   ____Min/Hr   Exercise_____

                                 Set/Reps   1.____   2.____   3.____

Tuesday_____   Month_____ Yr___

Exercise_____   **Exercise_____**   **Exercise_____**

   Weight   Reps   Weight   Reps   Weight   Reps

1.   X   1.   X   1.   X
2.   X   2.   X   2.   X
3.   X   3.   X   3.   X
4.   X   4.   X   4.   X
5.   X   5.   X   5.   X

Exercise_____   **Exercise_____**   **Exercise_____**

   Weight   Reps   Weight   Reps   Weight   Reps

1.   X   1.   X   1.   X
2.   X   2.   X   2.   X
3.   X   3.   X   3.   X
4.   X   4.   X   4.   X
5.   X   5.   X   5.   X

Exercise_____   **Exercise_____**   **Exercise_____**

   Weight   Reps   Weight   Reps   Weight   Reps

1.   X   1.   X   1.   X
2.   X   2.   X   2.   X
3.   X   3.   X   3.   X
4.   X   4.   X   4.   X
5.   X   5.   X   5.   X

Exercise_____   **Exercise_____**   **Exercise_____**

   Weight   Reps   Weight   Reps   Weight   Reps

1.   X   1.   X   1.   X
2.   X   2.   X   2.   X
3.   X   3.   X   3.   X
4.   X   4.   X   4.   X
5.   X   5.   X   5.   X

Aerobic Workout   **ABS**

Exercise   Time   Exercise_____

1._____   ____Min/Hr Set/Reps 1.____   2.____   3.____

2._____   ____Min/Hr Exercise_____

                                Set/Reps 1.____   2.____   3.____

Wednesday_____   Month____ Yr___

Exercise_____   **Exercise**_____   **Exercise**_____

  Weight   Reps   Weight   Reps   Weight   Reps

1.   X   1.   X   1.   X
2.   X   2.   X   2.   X
3.   X   3.   X   3.   X
4.   X   4.   X   4.   X
5.   X   5.   X   5.   X

Exercise_____   **Exercise**_____   **Exercise**_____

  Weight   Reps   Weight   Reps   Weight   Reps

1.   X   1.   X   1.   X
2.   X   2.   X   2.   X
3.   X   3.   X   3.   X
4.   X   4.   X   4.   X
5.   X   5.   X   5.   X

Exercise_____   **Exercise**_____   **Exercise**_____

  Weight   Reps   Weight   Reps   Weight   Reps

1.   X   1.   X   1.   X
2.   X   2.   X   2.   X
3.   X   3.   X   3.   X
4.   X   4.   X   4.   X
5.   X   5.   X   5.   X

Exercise_____   **Exercise**_____   **Exercise**_____

  Weight   Reps   Weight   Reps   Weight   Reps

1.   X   1.   X   1.   X
2.   X   2.   X   2.   X
3.   X   3.   X   3.   X
4.   X   4.   X   4.   X
5.   X   5.   X   5.   X

Aerobic Workout   **ABS**

Exercise   Time   Exercise_____

1._____   ____Min/Hr   Set/Reps 1.____   2.____   3.____

2._____   ____Min/Hr   Exercise_____

                                Set/Reps 1.____   2.____   3.____

Thursday_____   Month____ Yr___

Exercise_____   **Exercise_____**   **Exercise_____**

   Weight   Reps   Weight   Reps   Weight   Reps

1.   X   1.   X   1.   X
2.   X   2.   X   2.   X
3.   X   3.   X   3.   X
4.   X   4.   X   4.   X
5.   X   5.   X   5.   X

Exercise_____   **Exercise_____**   **Exercise_____**

   Weight   Reps   Weight   Reps   Weight   Reps

1.   X   1.   X   1.   X
2.   X   2.   X   2.   X
3.   X   3.   X   3.   X
4.   X   4.   X   4.   X
5.   X   5.   X   5.   X

Exercise_____   **Exercise_____**   **Exercise_____**

   Weight   Reps   Weight   Reps   Weight   Reps

1.   X   1.   X   1.   X
2.   X   2.   X   2.   X
3.   X   3.   X   3.   X
4.   X   4.   X   4.   X
5.   X   5.   X   5.   X

Exercise_____   **Exercise_____**   **Exercise_____**

   Weight   Reps   Weight   Reps   Weight   Reps

1.   X   1.   X   1.   X
2.   X   2.   X   2.   X
3.   X   3.   X   3.   X
4.   X   4.   X   4.   X
5.   X   5.   X   5.   X

Aerobic Workout   **ABS**

Exercise   Time   Exercise_____

1._____   ____Min/Hr Set/Reps 1.____   2.____   3.____

2._____   ____Min/Hr Exercise_____

                               Set/Reps 1.____   2.____   3.____

Friday_____   Month_____ Yr___

Exercise_____   **Exercise_____**   **Exercise_____**

  Weight   Reps   Weight   Reps   Weight   Reps

1.   X   1.   X   1.   X
2.   X   2.   X   2.   X
3.   X   3.   X   3.   X
4.   X   4.   X   4.   X
5.   X   5.   X   5.   X

Exercise_____   **Exercise_____**   **Exercise_____**

  Weight   Reps   Weight   Reps   Weight   Reps

1.   X   1.   X   1.   X
2.   X   2.   X   2.   X
3.   X   3.   X   3.   X
4.   X   4.   X   4.   X
5.   X   5.   X   5.   X

Exercise_____   **Exercise_____**   **Exercise_____**

  Weight   Reps   Weight   Reps   Weight   Reps

1.   X   1.   X   1.   X
2.   X   2.   X   2.   X
3.   X   3.   X   3.   X
4.   X   4.   X   4.   X
5.   X   5.   X   5.   X

Exercise_____   **Exercise_____**   **Exercise_____**

  Weight   Reps   Weight   Reps   Weight   Reps

1.   X   1.   X   1.   X
2.   X   2.   X   2.   X
3.   X   3.   X   3.   X
4.   X   4.   X   4.   X
5.   X   5.   X   5.   X

Aerobic Workout   **ABS**

Exercise   Time   Exercise_____

1._____ ____Min/Hr Set/Reps 1.____   2.____   3._____

2._____ ____Min/Hr Exercise_____

                              Set/Reps 1.____   2.____   3._____

Saturday_____   Month_____ Yr___

Exercise_____   **Exercise_____**   **Exercise_____**

   Weight   Reps   Weight   Reps   Weight   Reps

1.	X	1.	X	1.	X
2.	X	2.	X	2.	X
3.	X	3.	X	3.	X
4.	X	4.	X	4.	X
5.	X	5.	X	5.	X

Exercise_____   **Exercise_____**   **Exercise_____**

   Weight   Reps   Weight   Reps   Weight   Reps

1.	X	1.	X	1.	X
2.	X	2.	X	2.	X
3.	X	3.	X	3.	X
4.	X	4.	X	4.	X
5.	X	5.	X	5.	X

Exercise_____   **Exercise_____**   **Exercise_____**

   Weight   Reps   Weight   Reps   Weight   Reps

1.	X	1.	X	1.	X
2.	X	2.	X	2.	X
3.	X	3.	X	3.	X
4.	X	4.	X	4.	X
5.	X	5.	X	5.	X

Exercise_____   **Exercise_____**   **Exercise_____**

   Weight   Reps   Weight   Reps   Weight   Reps

1.	X	1.	X	1.	X
2.	X	2.	X	2.	X
3.	X	3.	X	3.	X
4.	X	4.	X	4.	X
5.	X	5.	X	5.	X

Aerobic Workout   **ABS**

Exercise   Time   Exercise_____

1._____ ____Min/Hr   Set/Reps   1.____   2.____   3.____

2._____ ____Min/Hr   Exercise_____

                          Set/Reps   1.____   2.____   3.____

Notes

Sunday_____   Month____ Yr___

Exercise_____   **Exercise_____**   **Exercise_____**

   Weight   Reps   Weight   Reps   Weight   Reps

1.   X   1.   X   1.   X
2.   X   2.   X   2.   X
3.   X   3.   X   3.   X
4.   X   4.   X   4.   X
5.   X   5.   X   5.   X

Exercise_____   **Exercise_____**   **Exercise_____**

   Weight   Reps   Weight   Reps   Weight   Reps

1.   X   1.   X   1.   X
2.   X   2.   X   2.   X
3.   X   3.   X   3.   X
4.   X   4.   X   4.   X
5.   X   5.   X   5.   X

Exercise_____   **Exercise_____**   **Exercise_____**

   Weight   Reps   Weight   Reps   Weight   Reps

1.   X   1.   X   1.   X
2.   X   2.   X   2.   X
3.   X   3.   X   3.   X
4.   X   4.   X   4.   X
5.   X   5.   X   5.   X

Exercise_____   **Exercise_____**   **Exercise_____**

   Weight   Reps   Weight   Reps   Weight   Reps

1.   X   1.   X   1.   X
2.   X   2.   X   2.   X
3.   X   3.   X   3.   X
4.   X   4.   X   4.   X
5.   X   5.   X   5.   X

Aerobic Workout   **ABS**

Exercise   Time   Exercise_____

1._____   ____Min/Hr Set/Reps 1.____   2.____   3.____

2._____   ____Min/Hr Exercise_____

                               Set/Reps 1.____   2.____   3.____

Monday_____   Month_____ Yr___

Exercise_____   **Exercise_____**   **Exercise_____**

   Weight   Reps   Weight   Reps   Weight   Reps

1.   X   1.   X   1.   X
2.   X   2.   X   2.   X
3.   X   3.   X   3.   X
4.   X   4.   X   4.   X
5.   X   5.   X   5.   X

Exercise_____   **Exercise_____**   **Exercise_____**

   Weight   Reps   Weight   Reps   Weight   Reps

1.   X   1.   X   1.   X
2.   X   2.   X   2.   X
3.   X   3.   X   3.   X
4.   X   4.   X   4.   X
5.   X   5.   X   5.   X

Exercise_____   **Exercise_____**   **Exercise_____**

   Weight   Reps   Weight   Reps   Weight   Reps

1.   X   1.   X   1.   X
2.   X   2.   X   2.   X
3.   X   3.   X   3.   X
4.   X   4.   X   4.   X
5.   X   5.   X   5.   X

Exercise_____   **Exercise_____**   **Exercise_____**

   Weight   Reps   Weight   Reps   Weight   Reps

1.   X   1.   X   1.   X
2.   X   2.   X   2.   X
3.   X   3.   X   3.   X
4.   X   4.   X   4.   X
5.   X   5.   X   5.   X

Aerobic Workout   **ABS**

Exercise   Time   Exercise_____

1._____   ____Min/Hr   Set/Reps 1.____   2.____   3.____

2._____   ____Min/Hr   Exercise_____

                              Set/Reps 1.____   2.____   3.____

Tuesday_____   Month_____ Yr___

Exercise_____   **Exercise_____**   **Exercise_____**

  Weight   Reps   Weight   Reps   Weight   Reps

1.   X   1.   X   1.   X
2.   X   2.   X   2.   X
3.   X   3.   X   3.   X
4.   X   4.   X   4.   X
5.   X   5.   X   5.   X

Exercise_____   **Exercise_____**   **Exercise_____**

  Weight   Reps   Weight   Reps   Weight   Reps

1.   X   1.   X   1.   X
2.   X   2.   X   2.   X
3.   X   3.   X   3.   X
4.   X   4.   X   4.   X
5.   X   5.   X   5.   X

Exercise_____   **Exercise_____**   **Exercise_____**

  Weight   Reps   Weight   Reps   Weight   Reps

1.   X   1.   X   1.   X
2.   X   2.   X   2.   X
3.   X   3.   X   3.   X
4.   X   4.   X   4.   X
5.   X   5.   X   5.   X

Exercise_____   **Exercise_____**   **Exercise_____**

  Weight   Reps   Weight   Reps   Weight   Reps

1.   X   1.   X   1.   X
2.   X   2.   X   2.   X
3.   X   3.   X   3.   X
4.   X   4.   X   4.   X
5.   X   5.   X   5.   X

Aerobic Workout   **ABS**

Exercise   Time   Exercise_____

1._____   ____Min/Hr   Set/Reps   1.____   2.____   3.____

2._____   ____Min/Hr   Exercise_____

                              Set/Reps   1.____   2.____   3.____

Wednesday_____   Month_____ Yr___

Exercise_____   **Exercise_____**   **Exercise_____**

   Weight   Reps   Weight   Reps   Weight   Reps

1.	X	1.	X	1.	X
2.	X	2.	X	2.	X
3.	X	3.	X	3.	X
4.	X	4.	X	4.	X
5.	X	5.	X	5.	X

Exercise_____   **Exercise_____**   **Exercise_____**

   Weight   Reps   Weight   Reps   Weight   Reps

1.	X	1.	X	1.	X
2.	X	2.	X	2.	X
3.	X	3.	X	3.	X
4.	X	4.	X	4.	X
5.	X	5.	X	5.	X

Exercise_____   **Exercise_____**   **Exercise_____**

   Weight   Reps   Weight   Reps   Weight   Reps

1.	X	1.	X	1.	X
2.	X	2.	X	2.	X
3.	X	3.	X	3.	X
4.	X	4.	X	4.	X
5.	X	5.	X	5.	X

Exercise_____   **Exercise_____**   **Exercise_____**

   Weight   Reps   Weight   Reps   Weight   Reps

1.	X	1.	X	1.	X
2.	X	2.	X	2.	X
3.	X	3.	X	3.	X
4.	X	4.	X	4.	X
5.	X	5.	X	5.	X

Aerobic Workout   **ABS**

Exercise   Time   Exercise_____

1._____ ____Min/Hr Set/Reps 1.____ 2.____ 3.____

2._____ ____Min/Hr Exercise_____

                      Set/Reps 1.____ 2.____ 3.____

Thursday_____   Month_____ Yr___

Exercise_____ **Exercise**_____ **Exercise**_____

   Weight   Reps   Weight   Reps   Weight   Reps

1.   X   1.   X   1.   X
2.   X   2.   X   2.   X
3.   X   3.   X   3.   X
4.   X   4.   X   4.   X
5.   X   5.   X   5.   X

Exercise_____ **Exercise**_____ **Exercise**_____

   Weight   Reps   Weight   Reps   Weight   Reps

1.   X   1.   X   1.   X
2.   X   2.   X   2.   X
3.   X   3.   X   3.   X
4.   X   4.   X   4.   X
5.   X   5.   X   5.   X

Exercise_____ **Exercise**_____ **Exercise**_____

   Weight   Reps   Weight   Reps   Weight   Reps

1.   X   1.   X   1.   X
2.   X   2.   X   2.   X
3.   X   3.   X   3.   X
4.   X   4.   X   4.   X
5.   X   5.   X   5.   X

Exercise_____ **Exercise**_____ **Exercise**_____

   Weight   Reps   Weight   Reps   Weight   Reps

1.   X   1.   X   1.   X
2.   X   2.   X   2.   X
3.   X   3.   X   3.   X
4.   X   4.   X   4.   X
5.   X   5.   X   5.   X

Aerobic Workout   **ABS**

Exercise   Time   Exercise_____

1._____   ____Min/Hr Set/Reps 1.____   2._____   3.____

2._____   ____Min/Hr Exercise_____

                               Set/Reps 1.____   2._____   3.____

Friday_____   Month_____ Yr___

Exercise_____   **Exercise_____**   **Exercise_____**

   Weight   Reps   Weight   Reps   Weight   Reps

1.   X   1.   X   1.   X
2.   X   2.   X   2.   X
3.   X   3.   X   3.   X
4.   X   4.   X   4.   X
5.   X   5.   X   5.   X

Exercise_____   **Exercise_____**   **Exercise_____**

   Weight   Reps   Weight   Reps   Weight   Reps

1.   X   1.   X   1.   X
2.   X   2.   X   2.   X
3.   X   3.   X   3.   X
4.   X   4.   X   4.   X
5.   X   5.   X   5.   X

Exercise_____   **Exercise_____**   **Exercise_____**

   Weight   Reps   Weight   Reps   Weight   Reps

1.   X   1.   X   1.   X
2.   X   2.   X   2.   X
3.   X   3.   X   3.   X
4.   X   4.   X   4.   X
5.   X   5.   X   5.   X

Exercise_____   **Exercise_____**   **Exercise_____**

   Weight   Reps   Weight   Reps   Weight   Reps

1.   X   1.   X   1.   X
2.   X   2.   X   2.   X
3.   X   3.   X   3.   X
4.   X   4.   X   4.   X
5.   X   5.   X   5.   X

Aerobic Workout   **ABS**

Exercise   Time   Exercise_____

1._____   ____Min/Hr Set/Reps 1.____   2.____   3.____

2._____   ____Min/Hr Exercise_____

                                Set/Reps 1.____   2.____   3.____

Saturday_____   Month_____ Yr___

Exercise_____   **Exercise**_____   **Exercise**_____

   Weight   Reps   Weight   Reps   Weight   Reps

1.   X   1.   X   1.   X
2.   X   2.   X   2.   X
3.   X   3.   X   3.   X
4.   X   4.   X   4.   X
5.   X   5.   X   5.   X

Exercise_____   **Exercise**_____   **Exercise**_____

   Weight   Reps   Weight   Reps   Weight   Reps

1.   X   1.   X   1.   X
2.   X   2.   X   2.   X
3.   X   3.   X   3.   X
4.   X   4.   X   4.   X
5.   X   5.   X   5.   X

Exercise_____   **Exercise**_____   **Exercise**_____

   Weight   Reps   Weight   Reps   Weight   Reps

1.   X   1.   X   1.   X
2.   X   2.   X   2.   X
3.   X   3.   X   3.   X
4.   X   4.   X   4.   X
5.   X   5.   X   5.   X

Exercise_____   **Exercise**_____   **Exercise**_____

   Weight   Reps   Weight   Reps   Weight   Reps

1.   X   1.   X   1.   X
2.   X   2.   X   2.   X
3.   X   3.   X   3.   X
4.   X   4.   X   4.   X
5.   X   5.   X   5.   X

Aerobic Workout   **ABS**

Exercise   Time   Exercise_____

1._____   ____Min/Hr   Set/Reps 1.____   2.____   3.____

2._____   ____Min/Hr   Exercise_____

                               Set/Reps 1.____   2.____   3.____

Notes

_____

_____

_____

_____

_____

_____

_____

_____

_____

_____

_____

_____

_____

_____

_____

_____

_____

_____

Sunday_____   Month_____ Yr___

Exercise_____   **Exercise_____**   **Exercise_____**

   Weight   Reps   Weight   Reps   Weight   Reps

1.   X   1.   X   1.   X
2.   X   2.   X   2.   X
3.   X   3.   X   3.   X
4.   X   4.   X   4.   X
5.   X   5.   X   5.   X

Exercise_____   **Exercise_____**   **Exercise_____**

   Weight   Reps   Weight   Reps   Weight   Reps

1.   X   1.   X   1.   X
2.   X   2.   X   2.   X
3.   X   3.   X   3.   X
4.   X   4.   X   4.   X
5.   X   5.   X   5.   X

Exercise_____   **Exercise_____**   **Exercise_____**

   Weight   Reps   Weight   Reps   Weight   Reps

1.   X   1.   X   1.   X
2.   X   2.   X   2.   X
3.   X   3.   X   3.   X
4.   X   4.   X   4.   X
5.   X   5.   X   5.   X

Exercise_____   **Exercise_____**   **Exercise_____**

   Weight   Reps   Weight   Reps   Weight   Reps

1.   X   1.   X   1.   X
2.   X   2.   X   2.   X
3.   X   3.   X   3.   X
4.   X   4.   X   4.   X
5.   X   5.   X   5.   X

Aerobic Workout   **ABS**

Exercise   Time   Exercise_____

1._____   ____Min/Hr   Set/Reps 1.____   2.____   3.____

2._____   ____Min/Hr   Exercise_____

                                  Set/Reps 1.____   2.____   3.____

Monday_____   Month_____ Yr___

Exercise_____   **Exercise_____**   **Exercise_____**

   Weight   Reps   Weight   Reps   Weight   Reps

1.   X   1.   X   1.   X
2.   X   2.   X   2.   X
3.   X   3.   X   3.   X
4.   X   4.   X   4.   X
5.   X   5.   X   5.   X

Exercise_____   **Exercise_____**   **Exercise_____**

   Weight   Reps   Weight   Reps   Weight   Reps

1.   X   1.   X   1.   X
2.   X   2.   X   2.   X
3.   X   3.   X   3.   X
4.   X   4.   X   4.   X
5.   X   5.   X   5.   X

Exercise_____   **Exercise_____**   **Exercise_____**

   Weight   Reps   Weight   Reps   Weight   Reps

1.   X   1.   X   1.   X
2.   X   2.   X   2.   X
3.   X   3.   X   3.   X
4.   X   4.   X   4.   X
5.   X   5.   X   5.   X

Exercise_____   **Exercise_____**   **Exercise_____**

   Weight   Reps   Weight   Reps   Weight   Reps

1.   X   1.   X   1.   X
2.   X   2.   X   2.   X
3.   X   3.   X   3.   X
4.   X   4.   X   4.   X
5.   X   5.   X   5.   X

Aerobic Workout   **ABS**

Exercise   Time   Exercise_____

1._____ ____Min/Hr Set/Reps 1.____ 2.____ 3.____

2._____ ____Min/Hr Exercise_____

                         Set/Reps 1.____ 2.____ 3.____

Tuesday_____   Month_____ Yr___

Exercise_____   **Exercise**_____   **Exercise**_____

   Weight   Reps   Weight   Reps   Weight   Reps

1.	X	1.	X	1.	X
2.	X	2.	X	2.	X
3.	X	3.	X	3.	X
4.	X	4.	X	4.	X
5.	X	5.	X	5.	X

Exercise_____   **Exercise**_____   **Exercise**_____

   Weight   Reps   Weight   Reps   Weight   Reps

1.	X	1.	X	1.	X
2.	X	2.	X	2.	X
3.	X	3.	X	3.	X
4.	X	4.	X	4.	X
5.	X	5.	X	5.	X

Exercise_____   **Exercise**_____   **Exercise**_____

   Weight   Reps   Weight   Reps   Weight   Reps

1.	X	1.	X	1.	X
2.	X	2.	X	2.	X
3.	X	3.	X	3.	X
4.	X	4.	X	4.	X
5.	X	5.	X	5.	X

Exercise_____   **Exercise**_____   **Exercise**_____

   Weight   Reps   Weight   Reps   Weight   Reps

1.	X	1.	X	1.	X
2.	X	2.	X	2.	X
3.	X	3.	X	3.	X
4.	X	4.	X	4.	X
5.	X	5.	X	5.	X

Aerobic Workout   **ABS**

Exercise   Time   Exercise_____

1._____   ____Min/Hr   Set/Reps   1.____   2.____   3.____

2._____   ____Min/Hr   Exercise_____

                                   Set/Reps   1.____   2.____   3.____

Wednesday_____   Month_____ Yr___

Exercise_____   **Exercise_____**   **Exercise_____**

    Weight   Reps   Weight   Reps   Weight   Reps

1.   X   1.   X   1.   X
2.   X   2.   X   2.   X
3.   X   3.   X   3.   X
4.   X   4.   X   4.   X
5.   X   5.   X   5.   X

Exercise_____   **Exercise_____**   **Exercise_____**

    Weight   Reps   Weight   Reps   Weight   Reps

1.   X   1.   X   1.   X
2.   X   2.   X   2.   X
3.   X   3.   X   3.   X
4.   X   4.   X   4.   X
5.   X   5.   X   5.   X

Exercise_____   **Exercise_____**   **Exercise_____**

    Weight   Reps   Weight   Reps   Weight   Reps

1.   X   1.   X   1.   X
2.   X   2.   X   2.   X
3.   X   3.   X   3.   X
4.   X   4.   X   4.   X
5.   X   5.   X   5.   X

Exercise_____   **Exercise_____**   **Exercise_____**

    Weight   Reps   Weight   Reps   Weight   Reps

1.   X   1.   X   1.   X
2.   X   2.   X   2.   X
3.   X   3.   X   3.   X
4.   X   4.   X   4.   X
5.   X   5.   X   5.   X

Aerobic Workout   **ABS**

Exercise   Time   Exercise_____

1._____   ____Min/Hr Set/Reps 1.____   2.____   3.____

2._____   ____Min/Hr Exercise_____

                            Set/Reps 1.____   2.____   3.____

Thursday_____   Month____   Yr___

Exercise_____   **Exercise**_____   **Exercise**_____

Weight   Reps   Weight   Reps   Weight   Reps

1.   X   1.   X   1.   X
2.   X   2.   X   2.   X
3.   X   3.   X   3.   X
4.   X   4.   X   4.   X
5.   X   5.   X   5.   X

Exercise_____   **Exercise**_____   **Exercise**_____

Weight   Reps   Weight   Reps   Weight   Reps

1.   X   1.   X   1.   X
2.   X   2.   X   2.   X
3.   X   3.   X   3.   X
4.   X   4.   X   4.   X
5.   X   5.   X   5.   X

Exercise_____   **Exercise**_____   **Exercise**_____

Weight   Reps   Weight   Reps   Weight   Reps

1.   X   1.   X   1.   X
2.   X   2.   X   2.   X
3.   X   3.   X   3.   X
4.   X   4.   X   4.   X
5.   X   5.   X   5.   X

Exercise_____   **Exercise**_____   **Exercise**_____

Weight   Reps   Weight   Reps   Weight   Reps

1.   X   1.   X   1.   X
2.   X   2.   X   2.   X
3.   X   3.   X   3.   X
4.   X   4.   X   4.   X
5.   X   5.   X   5.   X

Aerobic Workout   **ABS**

Exercise   Time   Exercise_____

1._____   ____Min/Hr   Set/Reps   1.____   2.____   3.____

2._____   ____Min/Hr   Exercise_____

                              Set/Reps   1.____   2.____   3.____

Friday_____   Month_____ Yr___

Exercise_____   **Exercise**_____   **Exercise**_____

   Weight   Reps   Weight   Reps   Weight   Reps

1.   X   1.   X   1.   X
2.   X   2.   X   2.   X
3.   X   3.   X   3.   X
4.   X   4.   X   4.   X
5.   X   5.   X   5.   X

Exercise_____   **Exercise**_____   **Exercise**_____

   Weight   Reps   Weight   Reps   Weight   Reps

1.   X   1.   X   1.   X
2.   X   2.   X   2.   X
3.   X   3.   X   3.   X
4.   X   4.   X   4.   X
5.   X   5.   X   5.   X

Exercise_____   **Exercise**_____   **Exercise**_____

   Weight   Reps   Weight   Reps   Weight   Reps

1.   X   1.   X   1.   X
2.   X   2.   X   2.   X
3.   X   3.   X   3.   X
4.   X   4.   X   4.   X
5.   X   5.   X   5.   X

Exercise_____   **Exercise**_____   **Exercise**_____

   Weight   Reps   Weight   Reps   Weight   Reps

1.   X   1.   X   1.   X
2.   X   2.   X   2.   X
3.   X   3.   X   3.   X
4.   X   4.   X   4.   X
5.   X   5.   X   5.   X

Aerobic Workout   **ABS**

Exercise   Time   Exercise_____

1._____   ____Min/Hr Set/Reps 1.____   2.____   3.____

2._____   ____Min/Hr Exercise_____

                                Set/Reps 1.____   2.____   3.____

Saturday_____   Month_____ Yr___

Exercise_____   **Exercise_____**   **Exercise_____**

  Weight   Reps   Weight   Reps   Weight   Reps

1.   X   1.   X   1.   X
2.   X   2.   X   2.   X
3.   X   3.   X   3.   X
4.   X   4.   X   4.   X
5.   X   5.   X   5.   X

Exercise_____   **Exercise_____**   **Exercise_____**

  Weight   Reps   Weight   Reps   Weight   Reps

1.   X   1.   X   1.   X
2.   X   2.   X   2.   X
3.   X   3.   X   3.   X
4.   X   4.   X   4.   X
5.   X   5.   X   5.   X

Exercise_____   **Exercise_____**   **Exercise_____**

  Weight   Reps   Weight   Reps   Weight   Reps

1.   X   1.   X   1.   X
2.   X   2.   X   2.   X
3.   X   3.   X   3.   X
4.   X   4.   X   4.   X
5.   X   5.   X   5.   X

Exercise_____   **Exercise_____**   **Exercise_____**

  Weight   Reps   Weight   Reps   Weight   Reps

1.   X   1.   X   1.   X
2.   X   2.   X   2.   X
3.   X   3.   X   3.   X
4.   X   4.   X   4.   X
5.   X   5.   X   5.   X

Aerobic Workout   **ABS**

Exercise   Time   Exercise_____

1._____   ____Min/Hr Set/Reps 1.____   2.____   3.____

2._____   ____Min/Hr Exercise_____

                        Set/Reps 1.____   2.____   3.____

Notes

MEAL PLANNER

Sunday _____   Month___   YR___

MEAL 1	CALORIES	CARBS	PROTEIN	FAT	SODIUM
	g	g	g	g	g
Time	g	g	g	g	g
:	g	g	g	g	g
	g	g	g	g	g

Total

MEAL 2	CALORIES	CARBS	PROTEIN	FAT	SODIUM
	g	g	g	g	g
Time	g	g	g	g	g
:	g	g	g	g	g
	g	g	g	g	g

Total

MEAL 3	CALORIES	CARBS	PROTEIN	FAT	SODIUM
	g	g	g	g	g
Time	g	g	g	g	g
:	g	g	g	g	g
	g	g	g	g	g

Total

MEAL 4	CALORIES	CARBS	PROTEIN	FAT	SODIUM
	g	g	g	g	g
Time	g	g	g	g	g
:	g	g	g	g	g
	g	g	g	g	g

Total

MEAL 5	CALORIES	CARBS	PROTEIN	FAT	SODIUM
	g	g	g	g	g
Time	g	g	g	g	g
:	g	g	g	g	g
	g	g	g	g	g

Total

Monday _____   Month____   YR____

MEAL 1	CALORIES	CARBS	PROTEIN	FAT	SODIUM
	g	g	g	g	g
Time	g	g	g	g	g
:	g	g	g	g	g
	g	g	g	g	g

Total

MEAL 2	CALORIES	CARBS	PROTEIN	FAT	SODIUM
	g	g	g	g	g
Time	g	g	g	g	g
:	g	g	g	g	g
	g	g	g	g	g

Total

MEAL 3	CALORIES	CARBS	PROTEIN	FAT	SODIUM
	g	g	g	g	g
Time	g	g	g	g	g
:	g	g	g	g	g
	g	g	g	g	g

Total

MEAL 4	CALORIES	CARBS	PROTEIN	FAT	SODIUM
	g	g	g	g	g
Time	g	g	g	g	g
:	g	g	g	g	g
	g	g	g	g	g

Total

MEAL 5	CALORIES	CARBS	PROTEIN	FAT	SODIUM
	g	g	g	g	g
Time	g	g	g	g	g
:	g	g	g	g	g
	g	g	g	g	g

Total

Tuesday _____   Month___   YR___

MEAL 1 <u>CALORIES</u> <u>CARBS</u>   <u>PROTEIN</u>   <u>FAT</u>   <u>SODIUM</u>

	CALORIES	CARBS	PROTEIN	FAT	SODIUM
	g	g	g	g	g
Time	g	g	g	g	g
:	g	g	g	g	g
	g	g	g	g	g

Total

MEAL 2 <u>CALORIES</u> <u>CARBS</u>   <u>PROTEIN</u>   <u>FAT</u>   <u>SODIUM</u>

	CALORIES	CARBS	PROTEIN	FAT	SODIUM
	g	g	g	g	g
Time	g	g	g	g	g
:	g	g	g	g	g
	g	g	g	g	g

Total

MEAL 3 <u>CALORIES</u> <u>CARBS</u>   <u>PROTEIN</u>   <u>FAT</u>   <u>SODIUM</u>

	CALORIES	CARBS	PROTEIN	FAT	SODIUM
	g	g	g	g	g
Time	g	g	g	g	g
:	g	g	g	g	g
	g	g	g	g	g

Total

MEAL 4 <u>CALORIES</u> <u>CARBS</u>   <u>PROTEIN</u>   <u>FAT</u>   <u>SODIUM</u>

	CALORIES	CARBS	PROTEIN	FAT	SODIUM
	g	g	g	g	g
Time	g	g	g	g	g
:	g	g	g	g	g
	g	g	g	g	g

Total

MEAL 5 <u>CALORIES</u> <u>CARBS</u>   <u>PROTEIN</u>   <u>FAT</u>   <u>SODIUM</u>

	CALORIES	CARBS	PROTEIN	FAT	SODIUM
	g	g	g	g	g
Time	g	g	g	g	g
:	g	g	g	g	g
	g	g	g	g	g

Total

Wednesday _____   Month___ YR___

MEAL 1 <u>CALORIES</u> <u>CARBS</u> <u>PROTEIN</u> <u>FAT</u> <u>SODIUM</u>
	g	g	g	g	g
Time	g	g	g	g	g
:	g	g	g	g	g
	g	g	g	g	g

Total

MEAL 2 <u>CALORIES</u> <u>CARBS</u> <u>PROTEIN</u> <u>FAT</u> <u>SODIUM</u>
	g	g	g	g	g
Time	g	g	g	g	g
:	g	g	g	g	g
	g	g	g	g	g

Total

MEAL 3 <u>CALORIES</u> <u>CARBS</u> <u>PROTEIN</u> <u>FAT</u> <u>SODIUM</u>
	g	g	g	g	g
Time	g	g	g	g	g
:	g	g	g	g	g
	g	g	g	g	g

Total

MEAL 4 <u>CALORIES</u> <u>CARBS</u> <u>PROTEIN</u> <u>FAT</u> <u>SODIUM</u>
	g	g	g	g	g
Time	g	g	g	g	g
:	g	g	g	g	g
	g	g	g	g	g

Total

MEAL 5 <u>CALORIES</u> <u>CARBS</u> <u>PROTEIN</u> <u>FAT</u> <u>SODIUM</u>
	g	g	g	g	g
Time	g	g	g	g	g
:	g	g	g	g	g
	g	g	g	g	g

Total

Thursday _____   Month___   YR___

MEAL 1 CALORIES	CARBS	PROTEIN	FAT	SODIUM
g	g	g	g	g
Time g	g	g	g	g
: g	g	g	g	g
g	g	g	g	g

Total

MEAL 2 CALORIES	CARBS	PROTEIN	FAT	SODIUM
g	g	g	g	g
Time g	g	g	g	g
: g	g	g	g	g
g	g	g	g	g

Total

MEAL 3 CALORIES	CARBS	PROTEIN	FAT	SODIUM
g	g	g	g	g
Time g	g	g	g	g
: g	g	g	g	g
g	g	g	g	g

Total

MEAL 4 CALORIES	CARBS	PROTEIN	FAT	SODIUM
g	g	g	g	g
Time g	g	g	g	g
: g	g	g	g	g
g	g	g	g	g

Total

MEAL 5 CALORIES	CARBS	PROTEIN	FAT	SODIUM
g	g	g	g	g
Time g	g	g	g	g
: g	g	g	g	g
g	g	g	g	g

Total

Friday _____   Month___   YR___

MEAL 1	CALORIES	CARBS	PROTEIN	FAT	SODIUM
	g	g	g	g	g
Time	g	g	g	g	g
:	g	g	g	g	g
	g	g	g	g	g

Total

MEAL 2	CALORIES	CARBS	PROTEIN	FAT	SODIUM
	g	g	g	g	g
Time	g	g	g	g	g
:	g	g	g	g	g
	g	g	g	g	g

Total

MEAL 3	CALORIES	CARBS	PROTEIN	FAT	SODIUM
	g	g	g	g	g
Time	g	g	g	g	g
:	g	g	g	g	g
	g	g	g	g	g

Total

MEAL 4	CALORIES	CARBS	PROTEIN	FAT	SODIUM
	g	g	g	g	g
Time	g	g	g	g	g
:	g	g	g	g	g
	g	g	g	g	g

Total

MEAL 5	CALORIES	CARBS	PROTEIN	FAT	SODIUM
	g	g	g	g	g
Time	g	g	g	g	g
:	g	g	g	g	g
	g	g	g	g	g

Total

Saturday _____   Month___   YR___

MEAL 1 <u>CALORIES</u> <u>CARBS</u> <u>PROTEIN</u> <u>FAT</u> <u>SODIUM</u>

	g	g	g	g	g
Time	g	g	g	g	g
:	g	g	g	g	g
	g	g	g	g	g

Total

MEAL 2 <u>CALORIES</u> <u>CARBS</u> <u>PROTEIN</u> <u>FAT</u> <u>SODIUM</u>

	g	g	g	g	g
Time	g	g	g	g	g
:	g	g	g	g	g
	g	g	g	g	g

Total

MEAL 3 <u>CALORIES</u> <u>CARBS</u> <u>PROTEIN</u> <u>FAT</u> <u>SODIUM</u>

	g	g	g	g	g
Time	g	g	g	g	g
:	g	g	g	g	g
	g	g	g	g	g

Total

MEAL 4 <u>CALORIES</u> <u>CARBS</u> <u>PROTEIN</u> <u>FAT</u> <u>SODIUM</u>

	g	g	g	g	g
Time	g	g	g	g	g
:	g	g	g	g	g
	g	g	g	g	g

Total

MEAL 5 <u>CALORIES</u> <u>CARBS</u> <u>PROTEIN</u> <u>FAT</u> <u>SODIUM</u>

	g	g	g	g	g
Time	g	g	g	g	g
:	g	g	g	g	g
	g	g	g	g	g

Total

Notes

_____

_____

_____

_____

_____

_____

_____

_____

_____

_____

_____

_____

_____

_____

_____

_____

_____

Sunday _____   Month___   YR___

MEAL 1	CALORIES	CARBS	PROTEIN	FAT	SODIUM
	g	g	g	g	g
Time	g	g	g	g	g
:	g	g	g	g	g
	g	g	g	g	g

Total

MEAL 2	CALORIES	CARBS	PROTEIN	FAT	SODIUM
	g	g	g	g	g
Time	g	g	g	g	g
:	g	g	g	g	g
	g	g	g	g	g

Total

MEAL 3	CALORIES	CARBS	PROTEIN	FAT	SODIUM
	g	g	g	g	g
Time	g	g	g	g	g
:	g	g	g	g	g
	g	g	g	g	g

Total

MEAL 4	CALORIES	CARBS	PROTEIN	FAT	SODIUM
	g	g	g	g	g
Time	g	g	g	g	g
:	g	g	g	g	g
	g	g	g	g	g

Total

MEAL 5	CALORIES	CARBS	PROTEIN	FAT	SODIUM
	g	g	g	g	g
Time	g	g	g	g	g
:	g	g	g	g	g
	g	g	g	g	g

Total

Monday _____   Month___ YR___

MEAL 1 <u>CALORIES</u> <u>CARBS</u> <u>PROTEIN</u> <u>FAT</u> <u>SODIUM</u>
	g	g	g	g	g
Time	g	g	g	g	g
:	g	g	g	g	g
	g	g	g	g	g

Total

MEAL 2 <u>CALORIES</u> <u>CARBS</u> <u>PROTEIN</u> <u>FAT</u> <u>SODIUM</u>
	g	g	g	g	g
Time	g	g	g	g	g
:	g	g	g	g	g
	g	g	g	g	g

Total

MEAL 3 <u>CALORIES</u> <u>CARBS</u> <u>PROTEIN</u> <u>FAT</u> <u>SODIUM</u>
	g	g	g	g	g
Time	g	g	g	g	g
:	g	g	g	g	g
	g	g	g	g	g

Total

MEAL 4 <u>CALORIES</u> <u>CARBS</u> <u>PROTEIN</u> <u>FAT</u> <u>SODIUM</u>
	g	g	g	g	g
Time	g	g	g	g	g
:	g	g	g	g	g
	g	g	g	g	g

Total

MEAL 5 <u>CALORIES</u> <u>CARBS</u> <u>PROTEIN</u> <u>FAT</u> <u>SODIUM</u>
	g	g	g	g	g
Time	g	g	g	g	g
:	g	g	g	g	g
	g	g	g	g	g

Total

Tuesday _____   Month___   YR___

MEAL 1	CALORIES	CARBS	PROTEIN	FAT	SODIUM
	g	g	g	g	g
Time	g	g	g	g	g
:	g	g	g	g	g
	g	g	g	g	g

Total

MEAL 2	CALORIES	CARBS	PROTEIN	FAT	SODIUM
	g	g	g	g	g
Time	g	g	g	g	g
:	g	g	g	g	g
	g	g	g	g	g

Total

MEAL 3	CALORIES	CARBS	PROTEIN	FAT	SODIUM
	g	g	g	g	g
Time	g	g	g	g	g
:	g	g	g	g	g
	g	g	g	g	g

Total

MEAL 4	CALORIES	CARBS	PROTEIN	FAT	SODIUM
	g	g	g	g	g
Time	g	g	g	g	g
:	g	g	g	g	g
	g	g	g	g	g

Total

MEAL 5	CALORIES	CARBS	PROTEIN	FAT	SODIUM
	g	g	g	g	g
Time	g	g	g	g	g
:	g	g	g	g	g
	g	g	g	g	g

Total

Wednesday _____   Month___   YR___

MEAL 1	CALORIES	CARBS	PROTEIN	FAT	SODIUM
	g	g	g	g	g
Time	g	g	g	g	g
:	g	g	g	g	g
	g	g	g	g	g

Total

MEAL 2	CALORIES	CARBS	PROTEIN	FAT	SODIUM
	g	g	g	g	g
Time	g	g	g	g	g
:	g	g	g	g	g
	g	g	g	g	g

Total

MEAL 3	CALORIES	CARBS	PROTEIN	FAT	SODIUM
	g	g	g	g	g
Time	g	g	g	g	g
:	g	g	g	g	g
	g	g	g	g	g

Total

MEAL 4	CALORIES	CARBS	PROTEIN	FAT	SODIUM
	g	g	g	g	g
Time	g	g	g	g	g
:	g	g	g	g	g
	g	g	g	g	g

Total

MEAL 5	CALORIES	CARBS	PROTEIN	FAT	SODIUM
	g	g	g	g	g
Time	g	g	g	g	g
:	g	g	g	g	g
	g	g	g	g	g

Total

Thursday _____   Month___   YR___

MEAL 1 <u>CALORIES</u> <u>CARBS</u> <u>PROTEIN</u> <u>FAT</u> <u>SODIUM</u>

	CALORIES	CARBS	PROTEIN	FAT	SODIUM
	g	g	g	g	g
Time	g	g	g	g	g
:	g	g	g	g	g
	g	g	g	g	g

Total

MEAL 2 <u>CALORIES</u> <u>CARBS</u> <u>PROTEIN</u> <u>FAT</u> <u>SODIUM</u>

	CALORIES	CARBS	PROTEIN	FAT	SODIUM
	g	g	g	g	g
Time	g	g	g	g	g
:	g	g	g	g	g
	g	g	g	g	g

Total

MEAL 3 <u>CALORIES</u> <u>CARBS</u> <u>PROTEIN</u> <u>FAT</u> <u>SODIUM</u>

	CALORIES	CARBS	PROTEIN	FAT	SODIUM
	g	g	g	g	g
Time	g	g	g	g	g
:	g	g	g	g	g
	g	g	g	g	g

Total

MEAL 4 <u>CALORIES</u> <u>CARBS</u> <u>PROTEIN</u> <u>FAT</u> <u>SODIUM</u>

	CALORIES	CARBS	PROTEIN	FAT	SODIUM
	g	g	g	g	g
Time	g	g	g	g	g
:	g	g	g	g	g
	g	g	g	g	g

Total

MEAL 5 <u>CALORIES</u> <u>CARBS</u> <u>PROTEIN</u> <u>FAT</u> <u>SODIUM</u>

	CALORIES	CARBS	PROTEIN	FAT	SODIUM
	g	g	g	g	g
Time	g	g	g	g	g
:	g	g	g	g	g
	g	g	g	g	g

Total

Friday _____   Month____   YR____

MEAL 1	CALORIES	CARBS	PROTEIN	FAT	SODIUM
	g	g	g	g	g
Time	g	g	g	g	g
:	g	g	g	g	g
	g	g	g	g	g

Total

MEAL 2	CALORIES	CARBS	PROTEIN	FAT	SODIUM
	g	g	g	g	g
Time	g	g	g	g	g
:	g	g	g	g	g
	g	g	g	g	g

Total

MEAL 3	CALORIES	CARBS	PROTEIN	FAT	SODIUM
	g	g	g	g	g
Time	g	g	g	g	g
:	g	g	g	g	g
	g	g	g	g	g

Total

MEAL 4	CALORIES	CARBS	PROTEIN	FAT	SODIUM
	g	g	g	g	g
Time	g	g	g	g	g
:	g	g	g	g	g
	g	g	g	g	g

Total

MEAL 5	CALORIES	CARBS	PROTEIN	FAT	SODIUM
	g	g	g	g	g
Time	g	g	g	g	g
:	g	g	g	g	g
	g	g	g	g	g

Total

Saturday _____   Month___   YR___

MEAL 1	CALORIES	CARBS	PROTEIN	FAT	SODIUM
	g	g	g	g	g
Time	g	g	g	g	g
:	g	g	g	g	g
	g	g	g	g	g

Total

MEAL 2	CALORIES	CARBS	PROTEIN	FAT	SODIUM
	g	g	g	g	g
Time	g	g	g	g	g
:	g	g	g	g	g
	g	g	g	g	g

Total

MEAL 3	CALORIES	CARBS	PROTEIN	FAT	SODIUM
	g	g	g	g	g
Time	g	g	g	g	g
:	g	g	g	g	g
	g	g	g	g	g

Total

MEAL 4	CALORIES	CARBS	PROTEIN	FAT	SODIUM
	g	g	g	g	g
Time	g	g	g	g	g
:	g	g	g	g	g
	g	g	g	g	g

Total

MEAL 5	CALORIES	CARBS	PROTEIN	FAT	SODIUM
	g	g	g	g	g
Time	g	g	g	g	g
:	g	g	g	g	g
	g	g	g	g	g

Total

Notes

_____

_____

_____

_____

_____

_____

_____

_____

_____

_____

_____

_____

_____

_____

_____

_____

_____

_____

Sunday _____   Month____   YR____

MEAL 1 <u>CALORIES</u>   <u>CARBS</u>   <u>PROTEIN</u>   <u>FAT</u>   <u>SODIUM</u>

	CALORIES	CARBS	PROTEIN	FAT	SODIUM
	g	g	g	g	g
Time	g	g	g	g	g
:	g	g	g	g	g
	g	g	g	g	g

Total

MEAL 2 <u>CALORIES</u>   <u>CARBS</u>   <u>PROTEIN</u>   <u>FAT</u>   <u>SODIUM</u>

	CALORIES	CARBS	PROTEIN	FAT	SODIUM
	g	g	g	g	g
Time	g	g	g	g	g
:	g	g	g	g	g
	g	g	g	g	g

Total

MEAL 3 <u>CALORIES</u>   <u>CARBS</u>   <u>PROTEIN</u>   <u>FAT</u>   <u>SODIUM</u>

	CALORIES	CARBS	PROTEIN	FAT	SODIUM
	g	g	g	g	g
Time	g	g	g	g	g
:	g	g	g	g	g
	g	g	g	g	g

Total

MEAL 4 <u>CALORIES</u>   <u>CARBS</u>   <u>PROTEIN</u>   <u>FAT</u>   <u>SODIUM</u>

	CALORIES	CARBS	PROTEIN	FAT	SODIUM
	g	g	g	g	g
Time	g	g	g	g	g
:	g	g	g	g	g
	g	g	g	g	g

Total

MEAL 5 <u>CALORIES</u>   <u>CARBS</u>   <u>PROTEIN</u>   <u>FAT</u>   <u>SODIUM</u>

	CALORIES	CARBS	PROTEIN	FAT	SODIUM
	g	g	g	g	g
Time	g	g	g	g	g
:	g	g	g	g	g
	g	g	g	g	g

Total

Monday _____   Month___   YR___

MEAL 1	CALORIES	CARBS	PROTEIN	FAT	SODIUM
	g	g	g	g	g
Time	g	g	g	g	g
:	g	g	g	g	g
	g	g	g	g	g

Total

MEAL 2	CALORIES	CARBS	PROTEIN	FAT	SODIUM
	g	g	g	g	g
Time	g	g	g	g	g
:	g	g	g	g	g
	g	g	g	g	g

Total

MEAL 3	CALORIES	CARBS	PROTEIN	FAT	SODIUM
	g	g	g	g	g
Time	g	g	g	g	g
:	g	g	g	g	g
	g	g	g	g	g

Total

MEAL 4	CALORIES	CARBS	PROTEIN	FAT	SODIUM
	g	g	g	g	g
Time	g	g	g	g	g
:	g	g	g	g	g
	g	g	g	g	g

Total

MEAL 5	CALORIES	CARBS	PROTEIN	FAT	SODIUM
	g	g	g	g	g
Time	g	g	g	g	g
:	g	g	g	g	g
	g	g	g	g	g

Total

Tuesday _____   Month___   YR___

MEAL 1 <u>CALORIES</u> <u>CARBS</u>   <u>PROTEIN</u>   <u>FAT</u>   <u>SODIUM</u>

	g	g	g	g	g
Time	g	g	g	g	g
:	g	g	g	g	g
	g	g	g	g	g

Total

MEAL 2 <u>CALORIES</u> <u>CARBS</u>   <u>PROTEIN</u>   <u>FAT</u>   <u>SODIUM</u>

	g	g	g	g	g
Time	g	g	g	g	g
:	g	g	g	g	g
	g	g	g	g	g

Total

MEAL 3 <u>CALORIES</u> <u>CARBS</u>   <u>PROTEIN</u>   <u>FAT</u>   <u>SODIUM</u>

	g	g	g	g	g
Time	g	g	g	g	g
:	g	g	g	g	g
	g	g	g	g	g

Total

MEAL 4 <u>CALORIES</u> <u>CARBS</u>   <u>PROTEIN</u>   <u>FAT</u>   <u>SODIUM</u>

	g	g	g	g	g
Time	g	g	g	g	g
:	g	g	g	g	g
	g	g	g	g	g

Total

MEAL 5 <u>CALORIES</u> <u>CARBS</u>   <u>PROTEIN</u>   <u>FAT</u>   <u>SODIUM</u>

	g	g	g	g	g
Time	g	g	g	g	g
:	g	g	g	g	g
	g	g	g	g	g

Total

Wednesday _____   Month___   YR___

MEAL 1 <u>CALORIES</u>   <u>CARBS</u>   <u>PROTEIN</u>   <u>FAT</u>   <u>SODIUM</u>

	g	g	g	g	g
Time	g	g	g	g	g
:	g	g	g	g	g
	g	g	g	g	g

Total

MEAL 2 <u>CALORIES</u>   <u>CARBS</u>   <u>PROTEIN</u>   <u>FAT</u>   <u>SODIUM</u>

	g	g	g	g	g
Time	g	g	g	g	g
:	g	g	g	g	g
	g	g	g	g	g

Total

MEAL 3 <u>CALORIES</u>   <u>CARBS</u>   <u>PROTEIN</u>   <u>FAT</u>   <u>SODIUM</u>

	g	g	g	g	g
Time	g	g	g	g	g
:	g	g	g	g	g
	g	g	g	g	g

Total

MEAL 4 <u>CALORIES</u>   <u>CARBS</u>   <u>PROTEIN</u>   <u>FAT</u>   <u>SODIUM</u>

	g	g	g	g	g
Time	g	g	g	g	g
:	g	g	g	g	g
	g	g	g	g	g

Total

MEAL 5 <u>CALORIES</u>   <u>CARBS</u>   <u>PROTEIN</u>   <u>FAT</u>   <u>SODIUM</u>

	g	g	g	g	g
Time	g	g	g	g	g
:	g	g	g	g	g
	g	g	g	g	g

Total

Thursday _____   Month___   YR___

MEAL 1 <u>CALORIES</u>   <u>CARBS</u>   <u>PROTEIN</u>   <u>FAT</u>   <u>SODIUM</u>
            g   g   g   g   g
Time   g   g   g   g   g
:   g   g   g   g   g
            g   g   g   g   g

Total

MEAL 2 <u>CALORIES</u>   <u>CARBS</u>   <u>PROTEIN</u>   <u>FAT</u>   <u>SODIUM</u>
            g   g   g   g   g
Time   g   g   g   g   g
:   g   g   g   g   g
            g   g   g   g   g

Total

MEAL 3 <u>CALORIES</u>   <u>CARBS</u>   <u>PROTEIN</u>   <u>FAT</u>   <u>SODIUM</u>
            g   g   g   g   g
Time   g   g   g   g   g
:   g   g   g   g   g
            g   g   g   g   g

Total

MEAL 4 <u>CALORIES</u>   <u>CARBS</u>   <u>PROTEIN</u>   <u>FAT</u>   <u>SODIUM</u>
            g   g   g   g   g
Time   g   g   g   g   g
:   g   g   g   g   g
            g   g   g   g   g

Total

MEAL 5 <u>CALORIES</u>   <u>CARBS</u>   <u>PROTEIN</u>   <u>FAT</u>   <u>SODIUM</u>
            g   g   g   g   g
Time   g   g   g   g   g
:   g   g   g   g   g
            g   g   g   g   g

Total

Friday _____   Month___   YR___

MEAL 1	CALORIES	CARBS	PROTEIN	FAT	SODIUM
	g	g	g	g	g
Time	g	g	g	g	g
:	g	g	g	g	g
	g	g	g	g	g

Total

MEAL 2	CALORIES	CARBS	PROTEIN	FAT	SODIUM
	g	g	g	g	g
Time	g	g	g	g	g
:	g	g	g	g	g
	g	g	g	g	g

Total

MEAL 3	CALORIES	CARBS	PROTEIN	FAT	SODIUM
	g	g	g	g	g
Time	g	g	g	g	g
:	g	g	g	g	g
	g	g	g	g	g

Total

MEAL 4	CALORIES	CARBS	PROTEIN	FAT	SODIUM
	g	g	g	g	g
Time	g	g	g	g	g
:	g	g	g	g	g
	g	g	g	g	g

Total

MEAL 5	CALORIES	CARBS	PROTEIN	FAT	SODIUM
	g	g	g	g	g
Time	g	g	g	g	g
:	g	g	g	g	g
	g	g	g	g	g

Total

Saturday _____   Month___ YR___

MEAL 1 <u>CALORIES</u> <u>CARBS</u> <u>PROTEIN</u> <u>FAT</u> <u>SODIUM</u>

	CALORIES	CARBS	PROTEIN	FAT	SODIUM
	g	g	g	g	g
Time	g	g	g	g	g
:	g	g	g	g	g
	g	g	g	g	g

Total

MEAL 2 <u>CALORIES</u> <u>CARBS</u> <u>PROTEIN</u> <u>FAT</u> <u>SODIUM</u>

	CALORIES	CARBS	PROTEIN	FAT	SODIUM
	g	g	g	g	g
Time	g	g	g	g	g
:	g	g	g	g	g
	g	g	g	g	g

Total

MEAL 3 <u>CALORIES</u> <u>CARBS</u> <u>PROTEIN</u> <u>FAT</u> <u>SODIUM</u>

	CALORIES	CARBS	PROTEIN	FAT	SODIUM
	g	g	g	g	g
Time	g	g	g	g	g
:	g	g	g	g	g
	g	g	g	g	g

Total

MEAL 4 <u>CALORIES</u> <u>CARBS</u> <u>PROTEIN</u> <u>FAT</u> <u>SODIUM</u>

	CALORIES	CARBS	PROTEIN	FAT	SODIUM
	g	g	g	g	g
Time	g	g	g	g	g
:	g	g	g	g	g
	g	g	g	g	g

Total

MEAL 5 <u>CALORIES</u> <u>CARBS</u> <u>PROTEIN</u> <u>FAT</u> <u>SODIUM</u>

	CALORIES	CARBS	PROTEIN	FAT	SODIUM
	g	g	g	g	g
Time	g	g	g	g	g
:	g	g	g	g	g
	g	g	g	g	g

Total

Notes

_____

_____

_____

_____

_____

_____

_____

_____

_____

_____

_____

_____

_____

_____

_____

_____

Sunday _____   Month___   YR___

MEAL 1	CALORIES	CARBS	PROTEIN	FAT	SODIUM
	g	g	g	g	g
Time	g	g	g	g	g
:	g	g	g	g	g
	g	g	g	g	g

Total

MEAL 2	CALORIES	CARBS	PROTEIN	FAT	SODIUM
	g	g	g	g	g
Time	g	g	g	g	g
:	g	g	g	g	g
	g	g	g	g	g

Total

MEAL 3	CALORIES	CARBS	PROTEIN	FAT	SODIUM
	g	g	g	g	g
Time	g	g	g	g	g
:	g	g	g	g	g
	g	g	g	g	g

Total

MEAL 4	CALORIES	CARBS	PROTEIN	FAT	SODIUM
	g	g	g	g	g
Time	g	g	g	g	g
:	g	g	g	g	g
	g	g	g	g	g

Total

MEAL 5	CALORIES	CARBS	PROTEIN	FAT	SODIUM
	g	g	g	g	g
Time	g	g	g	g	g
:	g	g	g	g	g
	g	g	g	g	g

Total

Monday _____   Month___ YR___

MEAL 1	CALORIES	CARBS	PROTEIN	FAT	SODIUM
	g	g	g	g	g
Time	g	g	g	g	g
:	g	g	g	g	g
	g	g	g	g	g

Total

MEAL 2	CALORIES	CARBS	PROTEIN	FAT	SODIUM
	g	g	g	g	g
Time	g	g	g	g	g
:	g	g	g	g	g
	g	g	g	g	g

Total

MEAL 3	CALORIES	CARBS	PROTEIN	FAT	SODIUM
	g	g	g	g	g
Time	g	g	g	g	g
:	g	g	g	g	g
	g	g	g	g	g

Total

MEAL 4	CALORIES	CARBS	PROTEIN	FAT	SODIUM
	g	g	g	g	g
Time	g	g	g	g	g
:	g	g	g	g	g
	g	g	g	g	g

Total

MEAL 5	CALORIES	CARBS	PROTEIN	FAT	SODIUM
	g	g	g	g	g
Time	g	g	g	g	g
:	g	g	g	g	g
	g	g	g	g	g

Total

Tuesday _____   Month___   YR___

MEAL 1 <u>CALORIES</u>   <u>CARBS</u>   <u>PROTEIN</u>   <u>FAT</u>   <u>SODIUM</u>

	g	g	g	g	g
Time	g	g	g	g	g
:	g	g	g	g	g
	g	g	g	g	g

Total

MEAL 2 <u>CALORIES</u>   <u>CARBS</u>   <u>PROTEIN</u>   <u>FAT</u>   <u>SODIUM</u>

	g	g	g	g	g
Time	g	g	g	g	g
:	g	g	g	g	g
	g	g	g	g	g

Total

MEAL 3 <u>CALORIES</u>   <u>CARBS</u>   <u>PROTEIN</u>   <u>FAT</u>   <u>SODIUM</u>

	g	g	g	g	g
Time	g	g	g	g	g
:	g	g	g	g	g
	g	g	g	g	g

Total

MEAL 4 <u>CALORIES</u>   <u>CARBS</u>   <u>PROTEIN</u>   <u>FAT</u>   <u>SODIUM</u>

	g	g	g	g	g
Time	g	g	g	g	g
:	g	g	g	g	g
	g	g	g	g	g

Total

MEAL 5 <u>CALORIES</u>   <u>CARBS</u>   <u>PROTEIN</u>   <u>FAT</u>   <u>SODIUM</u>

	g	g	g	g	g
Time	g	g	g	g	g
:	g	g	g	g	g
	g	g	g	g	g

Total

Wednesday _____   Month___   YR___

MEAL 1	CALORIES	CARBS	PROTEIN	FAT	SODIUM
	g	g	g	g	g
Time	g	g	g	g	g
:	g	g	g	g	g
	g	g	g	g	g

Total

MEAL 2	CALORIES	CARBS	PROTEIN	FAT	SODIUM
	g	g	g	g	g
Time	g	g	g	g	g
:	g	g	g	g	g
	g	g	g	g	g

Total

MEAL 3	CALORIES	CARBS	PROTEIN	FAT	SODIUM
	g	g	g	g	g
Time	g	g	g	g	g
:	g	g	g	g	g
	g	g	g	g	g

Total

MEAL 4	CALORIES	CARBS	PROTEIN	FAT	SODIUM
	g	g	g	g	g
Time	g	g	g	g	g
:	g	g	g	g	g
	g	g	g	g	g

Total

MEAL 5	CALORIES	CARBS	PROTEIN	FAT	SODIUM
	g	g	g	g	g
Time	g	g	g	g	g
:	g	g	g	g	g
	g	g	g	g	g

Total

Thursday _____   Month___   YR___

MEAL 1	CALORIES	CARBS	PROTEIN	FAT	SODIUM
	g	g	g	g	g
Time	g	g	g	g	g
:	g	g	g	g	g
	g	g	g	g	g

Total

MEAL 2	CALORIES	CARBS	PROTEIN	FAT	SODIUM
	g	g	g	g	g
Time	g	g	g	g	g
:	g	g	g	g	g
	g	g	g	g	g

Total

MEAL 3	CALORIES	CARBS	PROTEIN	FAT	SODIUM
	g	g	g	g	g
Time	g	g	g	g	g
:	g	g	g	g	g
	g	g	g	g	g

Total

MEAL 4	CALORIES	CARBS	PROTEIN	FAT	SODIUM
	g	g	g	g	g
Time	g	g	g	g	g
:	g	g	g	g	g
	g	g	g	g	g

Total

MEAL 5	CALORIES	CARBS	PROTEIN	FAT	SODIUM
	g	g	g	g	g
Time	g	g	g	g	g
:	g	g	g	g	g
	g	g	g	g	g

Total

Friday _____   Month___   YR___

MEAL 1	CALORIES	CARBS	PROTEIN	FAT	SODIUM
	g	g	g	g	g
Time	g	g	g	g	g
:	g	g	g	g	g
	g	g	g	g	g

Total

MEAL 2	CALORIES	CARBS	PROTEIN	FAT	SODIUM
	g	g	g	g	g
Time	g	g	g	g	g
:	g	g	g	g	g
	g	g	g	g	g

Total

MEAL 3	CALORIES	CARBS	PROTEIN	FAT	SODIUM
	g	g	g	g	g
Time	g	g	g	g	g
:	g	g	g	g	g
	g	g	g	g	g

Total

MEAL 4	CALORIES	CARBS	PROTEIN	FAT	SODIUM
	g	g	g	g	g
Time	g	g	g	g	g
:	g	g	g	g	g
	g	g	g	g	g

Total

MEAL 5	CALORIES	CARBS	PROTEIN	FAT	SODIUM
	g	g	g	g	g
Time	g	g	g	g	g
:	g	g	g	g	g
	g	g	g	g	g

Total

Saturday _____   Month___   YR___

MEAL 1 <u>CALORIES</u> <u>CARBS</u> <u>PROTEIN</u> <u>FAT</u> <u>SODIUM</u>

	g	g	g	g	g
Time	g	g	g	g	g
:	g	g	g	g	g
	g	g	g	g	g

Total

MEAL 2 <u>CALORIES</u> <u>CARBS</u> <u>PROTEIN</u> <u>FAT</u> <u>SODIUM</u>

	g	g	g	g	g
Time	g	g	g	g	g
:	g	g	g	g	g
	g	g	g	g	g

Total

MEAL 3 <u>CALORIES</u> <u>CARBS</u> <u>PROTEIN</u> <u>FAT</u> <u>SODIUM</u>

	g	g	g	g	g
Time	g	g	g	g	g
:	g	g	g	g	g
	g	g	g	g	g

Total

MEAL 4 <u>CALORIES</u> <u>CARBS</u> <u>PROTEIN</u> <u>FAT</u> <u>SODIUM</u>

	g	g	g	g	g
Time	g	g	g	g	g
:	g	g	g	g	g
	g	g	g	g	g

Total

MEAL 5 <u>CALORIES</u> <u>CARBS</u> <u>PROTEIN</u> <u>FAT</u> <u>SODIUM</u>

	g	g	g	g	g
Time	g	g	g	g	g
:	g	g	g	g	g
	g	g	g	g	g

Total

Notes

Sunday _____   Month___   YR___

MEAL 1 <u>CALORIES</u>   <u>CARBS</u>   <u>PROTEIN</u>   <u>FAT</u>   <u>SODIUM</u>
	g	g	g	g	g
Time	g	g	g	g	g
:	g	g	g	g	g
	g	g	g	g	g

Total

MEAL 2 <u>CALORIES</u>   <u>CARBS</u>   <u>PROTEIN</u>   <u>FAT</u>   <u>SODIUM</u>
	g	g	g	g	g
Time	g	g	g	g	g
:	g	g	g	g	g
	g	g	g	g	g

Total

MEAL 3 <u>CALORIES</u>   <u>CARBS</u>   <u>PROTEIN</u>   <u>FAT</u>   <u>SODIUM</u>
	g	g	g	g	g
Time	g	g	g	g	g
:	g	g	g	g	g
	g	g	g	g	g

Total

MEAL 4 <u>CALORIES</u>   <u>CARBS</u>   <u>PROTEIN</u>   <u>FAT</u>   <u>SODIUM</u>
	g	g	g	g	g
Time	g	g	g	g	g
:	g	g	g	g	g
	g	g	g	g	g

Total

MEAL 5 <u>CALORIES</u>   <u>CARBS</u>   <u>PROTEIN</u>   <u>FAT</u>   <u>SODIUM</u>
	g	g	g	g	g
Time	g	g	g	g	g
:	g	g	g	g	g
	g	g	g	g	g

Total

Monday _____   Month___   YR___

MEAL 1 <u>CALORIES</u>   <u>CARBS</u>   <u>PROTEIN</u>   <u>FAT</u>   <u>SODIUM</u>
	g	g	g	g	g
Time	g	g	g	g	g
:	g	g	g	g	g
	g	g	g	g	g

Total

MEAL 2 <u>CALORIES</u>   <u>CARBS</u>   <u>PROTEIN</u>   <u>FAT</u>   <u>SODIUM</u>
	g	g	g	g	g
Time	g	g	g	g	g
:	g	g	g	g	g
	g	g	g	g	g

Total

MEAL 3 <u>CALORIES</u>   <u>CARBS</u>   <u>PROTEIN</u>   <u>FAT</u>   <u>SODIUM</u>
	g	g	g	g	g
Time	g	g	g	g	g
:	g	g	g	g	g
	g	g	g	g	g

Total

MEAL 4 <u>CALORIES</u>   <u>CARBS</u>   <u>PROTEIN</u>   <u>FAT</u>   <u>SODIUM</u>
	g	g	g	g	g
Time	g	g	g	g	g
:	g	g	g	g	g
	g	g	g	g	g

Total

MEAL 5 <u>CALORIES</u>   <u>CARBS</u>   <u>PROTEIN</u>   <u>FAT</u>   <u>SODIUM</u>
	g	g	g	g	g
Time	g	g	g	g	g
:	g	g	g	g	g
	g	g	g	g	g

Total

Tuesday _____   Month___   YR___

MEAL 1	CALORIES	CARBS	PROTEIN	FAT	SODIUM
	g	g	g	g	g
Time	g	g	g	g	g
:	g	g	g	g	g
	g	g	g	g	g

Total

MEAL 2	CALORIES	CARBS	PROTEIN	FAT	SODIUM
	g	g	g	g	g
Time	g	g	g	g	g
:	g	g	g	g	g
	g	g	g	g	g

Total

MEAL 3	CALORIES	CARBS	PROTEIN	FAT	SODIUM
	g	g	g	g	g
Time	g	g	g	g	g
:	g	g	g	g	g
	g	g	g	g	g

Total

MEAL 4	CALORIES	CARBS	PROTEIN	FAT	SODIUM
	g	g	g	g	g
Time	g	g	g	g	g
:	g	g	g	g	g
	g	g	g	g	g

Total

MEAL 5	CALORIES	CARBS	PROTEIN	FAT	SODIUM
	g	g	g	g	g
Time	g	g	g	g	g
:	g	g	g	g	g
	g	g	g	g	g

Total

Wednesday _____   Month___   YR___

MEAL 1 <u>CALORIES</u> <u>CARBS</u> <u>PROTEIN</u> <u>FAT</u> <u>SODIUM</u>
	g	g	g	g	g
Time	g	g	g	g	g
:	g	g	g	g	g
	g	g	g	g	g

Total

MEAL 2 <u>CALORIES</u> <u>CARBS</u> <u>PROTEIN</u> <u>FAT</u> <u>SODIUM</u>
	g	g	g	g	g
Time	g	g	g	g	g
:	g	g	g	g	g
	g	g	g	g	g

Total

MEAL 3 <u>CALORIES</u> <u>CARBS</u> <u>PROTEIN</u> <u>FAT</u> <u>SODIUM</u>
	g	g	g	g	g
Time	g	g	g	g	g
:	g	g	g	g	g
	g	g	g	g	g

Total

MEAL 4 <u>CALORIES</u> <u>CARBS</u> <u>PROTEIN</u> <u>FAT</u> <u>SODIUM</u>
	g	g	g	g	g
Time	g	g	g	g	g
:	g	g	g	g	g
	g	g	g	g	g

Total

MEAL 5 <u>CALORIES</u> <u>CARBS</u> <u>PROTEIN</u> <u>FAT</u> <u>SODIUM</u>
	g	g	g	g	g
Time	g	g	g	g	g
:	g	g	g	g	g
	g	g	g	g	g

Total

135

Thursday _____   Month___   YR___

MEAL 1	CALORIES	CARBS	PROTEIN	FAT	SODIUM
	g	g	g	g	g
Time	g	g	g	g	g
:	g	g	g	g	g
	g	g	g	g	g

Total

MEAL 2	CALORIES	CARBS	PROTEIN	FAT	SODIUM
	g	g	g	g	g
Time	g	g	g	g	g
:	g	g	g	g	g
	g	g	g	g	g

Total

MEAL 3	CALORIES	CARBS	PROTEIN	FAT	SODIUM
	g	g	g	g	g
Time	g	g	g	g	g
:	g	g	g	g	g
	g	g	g	g	g

Total

MEAL 4	CALORIES	CARBS	PROTEIN	FAT	SODIUM
	g	g	g	g	g
Time	g	g	g	g	g
:	g	g	g	g	g
	g	g	g	g	g

Total

MEAL 5	CALORIES	CARBS	PROTEIN	FAT	SODIUM
	g	g	g	g	g
Time	g	g	g	g	g
:	g	g	g	g	g
	g	g	g	g	g

Total

Friday _____   Month___   YR___

MEAL 1	CALORIES	CARBS	PROTEIN	FAT	SODIUM
	g	g	g	g	g
Time	g	g	g	g	g
:	g	g	g	g	g
	g	g	g	g	g

Total

MEAL 2	CALORIES	CARBS	PROTEIN	FAT	SODIUM
	g	g	g	g	g
Time	g	g	g	g	g
:	g	g	g	g	g
	g	g	g	g	g

Total

MEAL 3	CALORIES	CARBS	PROTEIN	FAT	SODIUM
	g	g	g	g	g
Time	g	g	g	g	g
:	g	g	g	g	g
	g	g	g	g	g

Total

MEAL 4	CALORIES	CARBS	PROTEIN	FAT	SODIUM
	g	g	g	g	g
Time	g	g	g	g	g
:	g	g	g	g	g
	g	g	g	g	g

Total

MEAL 5	CALORIES	CARBS	PROTEIN	FAT	SODIUM
	g	g	g	g	g
Time	g	g	g	g	g
:	g	g	g	g	g
	g	g	g	g	g

Total

Saturday _____   Month___   YR___

MEAL 1 <u>CALORIES</u> <u>CARBS</u>   <u>PROTEIN</u>   <u>FAT</u>   <u>SODIUM</u>

	CALORIES	CARBS	PROTEIN	FAT	SODIUM
	g	g	g	g	g
Time	g	g	g	g	g
:	g	g	g	g	g
	g	g	g	g	g

Total

MEAL 2 <u>CALORIES</u> <u>CARBS</u>   <u>PROTEIN</u>   <u>FAT</u>   <u>SODIUM</u>

	CALORIES	CARBS	PROTEIN	FAT	SODIUM
	g	g	g	g	g
Time	g	g	g	g	g
:	g	g	g	g	g
	g	g	g	g	g

Total

MEAL 3 <u>CALORIES</u> <u>CARBS</u>   <u>PROTEIN</u>   <u>FAT</u>   <u>SODIUM</u>

	CALORIES	CARBS	PROTEIN	FAT	SODIUM
	g	g	g	g	g
Time	g	g	g	g	g
:	g	g	g	g	g
	g	g	g	g	g

Total

MEAL 4 <u>CALORIES</u> <u>CARBS</u>   <u>PROTEIN</u>   <u>FAT</u>   <u>SODIUM</u>

	CALORIES	CARBS	PROTEIN	FAT	SODIUM
	g	g	g	g	g
Time	g	g	g	g	g
:	g	g	g	g	g
	g	g	g	g	g

Total

MEAL 5 <u>CALORIES</u> <u>CARBS</u>   <u>PROTEIN</u>   <u>FAT</u>   <u>SODIUM</u>

	CALORIES	CARBS	PROTEIN	FAT	SODIUM
	g	g	g	g	g
Time	g	g	g	g	g
:	g	g	g	g	g
	g	g	g	g	g

Total

Notes

_____

_____

_____

_____

_____

_____

_____

_____

_____

_____

_____

_____

_____

_____

_____

_____

_____

_____

Sunday _____   Month___   YR___

MEAL 1 <u>CALORIES</u>   <u>CARBS</u>   <u>PROTEIN</u>   <u>FAT</u>   <u>SODIUM</u>

	CALORIES	CARBS	PROTEIN	FAT	SODIUM
	g	g	g	g	g
Time	g	g	g	g	g
:	g	g	g	g	g
	g	g	g	g	g

Total

MEAL 2 <u>CALORIES</u>   <u>CARBS</u>   <u>PROTEIN</u>   <u>FAT</u>   <u>SODIUM</u>

	CALORIES	CARBS	PROTEIN	FAT	SODIUM
	g	g	g	g	g
Time	g	g	g	g	g
:	g	g	g	g	g
	g	g	g	g	g

Total

MEAL 3 <u>CALORIES</u>   <u>CARBS</u>   <u>PROTEIN</u>   <u>FAT</u>   <u>SODIUM</u>

	CALORIES	CARBS	PROTEIN	FAT	SODIUM
	g	g	g	g	g
Time	g	g	g	g	g
:	g	g	g	g	g
	g	g	g	g	g

Total

MEAL 4 <u>CALORIES</u>   <u>CARBS</u>   <u>PROTEIN</u>   <u>FAT</u>   <u>SODIUM</u>

	CALORIES	CARBS	PROTEIN	FAT	SODIUM
	g	g	g	g	g
Time	g	g	g	g	g
:	g	g	g	g	g
	g	g	g	g	g

Total

MEAL 5 <u>CALORIES</u>   <u>CARBS</u>   <u>PROTEIN</u>   <u>FAT</u>   <u>SODIUM</u>

	CALORIES	CARBS	PROTEIN	FAT	SODIUM
	g	g	g	g	g
Time	g	g	g	g	g
:	g	g	g	g	g
	g	g	g	g	g

Total

Monday _____   Month___   YR___

MEAL 1	CALORIES	CARBS	PROTEIN	FAT	SODIUM
	g	g	g	g	g
Time	g	g	g	g	g
:	g	g	g	g	g
	g	g	g	g	g

Total

MEAL 2	CALORIES	CARBS	PROTEIN	FAT	SODIUM
	g	g	g	g	g
Time	g	g	g	g	g
:	g	g	g	g	g
	g	g	g	g	g

Total

MEAL 3	CALORIES	CARBS	PROTEIN	FAT	SODIUM
	g	g	g	g	g
Time	g	g	g	g	g
:	g	g	g	g	g
	g	g	g	g	g

Total

MEAL 4	CALORIES	CARBS	PROTEIN	FAT	SODIUM
	g	g	g	g	g
Time	g	g	g	g	g
:	g	g	g	g	g
	g	g	g	g	g

Total

MEAL 5	CALORIES	CARBS	PROTEIN	FAT	SODIUM
	g	g	g	g	g
Time	g	g	g	g	g
:	g	g	g	g	g
	g	g	g	g	g

Total

Tuesday _____   Month___   YR___

MEAL 1 <u>CALORIES</u> <u>CARBS</u> <u>PROTEIN</u> <u>FAT</u> <u>SODIUM</u>

	g	g	g	g	g
Time	g	g	g	g	g
:	g	g	g	g	g
	g	g	g	g	g

Total

MEAL 2 <u>CALORIES</u> <u>CARBS</u> <u>PROTEIN</u> <u>FAT</u> <u>SODIUM</u>

	g	g	g	g	g
Time	g	g	g	g	g
:	g	g	g	g	g
	g	g	g	g	g

Total

MEAL 3 <u>CALORIES</u> <u>CARBS</u> <u>PROTEIN</u> <u>FAT</u> <u>SODIUM</u>

	g	g	g	g	g
Time	g	g	g	g	g
:	g	g	g	g	g
	g	g	g	g	g

Total

MEAL 4 <u>CALORIES</u> <u>CARBS</u> <u>PROTEIN</u> <u>FAT</u> <u>SODIUM</u>

	g	g	g	g	g
Time	g	g	g	g	g
:	g	g	g	g	g
	g	g	g	g	g

Total

MEAL 5 <u>CALORIES</u> <u>CARBS</u> <u>PROTEIN</u> <u>FAT</u> <u>SODIUM</u>

	g	g	g	g	g
Time	g	g	g	g	g
:	g	g	g	g	g
	g	g	g	g	g

Total

Wednesday _____   Month___   YR___

MEAL 1	CALORIES	CARBS	PROTEIN	FAT	SODIUM
	g	g	g	g	g
Time	g	g	g	g	g
:	g	g	g	g	g
	g	g	g	g	g

Total

MEAL 2	CALORIES	CARBS	PROTEIN	FAT	SODIUM
	g	g	g	g	g
Time	g	g	g	g	g
:	g	g	g	g	g
	g	g	g	g	g

Total

MEAL 3	CALORIES	CARBS	PROTEIN	FAT	SODIUM
	g	g	g	g	g
Time	g	g	g	g	g
:	g	g	g	g	g
	g	g	g	g	g

Total

MEAL 4	CALORIES	CARBS	PROTEIN	FAT	SODIUM
	g	g	g	g	g
Time	g	g	g	g	g
:	g	g	g	g	g
	g	g	g	g	g

Total

MEAL 5	CALORIES	CARBS	PROTEIN	FAT	SODIUM
	g	g	g	g	g
Time	g	g	g	g	g
:	g	g	g	g	g
	g	g	g	g	g

Total

Thursday _____   Month___   YR___

MEAL 1	CALORIES	CARBS	PROTEIN	FAT	SODIUM
	g	g	g	g	g
Time	g	g	g	g	g
:	g	g	g	g	g
	g	g	g	g	g

Total

MEAL 2	CALORIES	CARBS	PROTEIN	FAT	SODIUM
	g	g	g	g	g
Time	g	g	g	g	g
:	g	g	g	g	g
	g	g	g	g	g

Total

MEAL 3	CALORIES	CARBS	PROTEIN	FAT	SODIUM
	g	g	g	g	g
Time	g	g	g	g	g
:	g	g	g	g	g
	g	g	g	g	g

Total

MEAL 4	CALORIES	CARBS	PROTEIN	FAT	SODIUM
	g	g	g	g	g
Time	g	g	g	g	g
:	g	g	g	g	g
	g	g	g	g	g

Total

MEAL 5	CALORIES	CARBS	PROTEIN	FAT	SODIUM
	g	g	g	g	g
Time	g	g	g	g	g
:	g	g	g	g	g
	g	g	g	g	g

Total

Friday _____   Month___   YR___

MEAL 1	CALORIES	CARBS	PROTEIN	FAT	SODIUM
	g	g	g	g	g
Time	g	g	g	g	g
:	g	g	g	g	g
	g	g	g	g	g

Total

MEAL 2	CALORIES	CARBS	PROTEIN	FAT	SODIUM
	g	g	g	g	g
Time	g	g	g	g	g
:	g	g	g	g	g
	g	g	g	g	g

Total

MEAL 3	CALORIES	CARBS	PROTEIN	FAT	SODIUM
	g	g	g	g	g
Time	g	g	g	g	g
:	g	g	g	g	g
	g	g	g	g	g

Total

MEAL 4	CALORIES	CARBS	PROTEIN	FAT	SODIUM
	g	g	g	g	g
Time	g	g	g	g	g
:	g	g	g	g	g
	g	g	g	g	g

Total

MEAL 5	CALORIES	CARBS	PROTEIN	FAT	SODIUM
	g	g	g	g	g
Time	g	g	g	g	g
:	g	g	g	g	g
	g	g	g	g	g

Total

Saturday _____   Month___ YR___

MEAL 1	CALORIES	CARBS	PROTEIN	FAT	SODIUM
	g	g	g	g	g
Time	g	g	g	g	g
:	g	g	g	g	g
	g	g	g	g	g

Total

MEAL 2	CALORIES	CARBS	PROTEIN	FAT	SODIUM
	g	g	g	g	g
Time	g	g	g	g	g
:	g	g	g	g	g
	g	g	g	g	g

Total

MEAL 3	CALORIES	CARBS	PROTEIN	FAT	SODIUM
	g	g	g	g	g
Time	g	g	g	g	g
:	g	g	g	g	g
	g	g	g	g	g

Total

MEAL 4	CALORIES	CARBS	PROTEIN	FAT	SODIUM
	g	g	g	g	g
Time	g	g	g	g	g
:	g	g	g	g	g
	g	g	g	g	g

Total

MEAL 5	CALORIES	CARBS	PROTEIN	FAT	SODIUM
	g	g	g	g	g
Time	g	g	g	g	g
:	g	g	g	g	g
	g	g	g	g	g

Total

Notes

Sunday _____   Month___   YR___

MEAL 1 CALORIES   CARBS   PROTEIN   FAT   SODIUM

	g	g	g	g	g
Time	g	g	g	g	g
:	g	g	g	g	g
	g	g	g	g	g

Total

MEAL 2 CALORIES   CARBS   PROTEIN   FAT   SODIUM

	g	g	g	g	g
Time	g	g	g	g	g
:	g	g	g	g	g
	g	g	g	g	g

Total

MEAL 3 CALORIES   CARBS   PROTEIN   FAT   SODIUM

	g	g	g	g	g
Time	g	g	g	g	g
:	g	g	g	g	g
	g	g	g	g	g

Total

MEAL 4 CALORIES   CARBS   PROTEIN   FAT   SODIUM

	g	g	g	g	g
Time	g	g	g	g	g
:	g	g	g	g	g
	g	g	g	g	g

Total

MEAL 5 CALORIES   CARBS   PROTEIN   FAT   SODIUM

	g	g	g	g	g
Time	g	g	g	g	g
:	g	g	g	g	g
	g	g	g	g	g

Total

Monday _____   Month___   YR___

MEAL 1	CALORIES	CARBS	PROTEIN	FAT	SODIUM
	g	g	g	g	g
Time	g	g	g	g	g
:	g	g	g	g	g
	g	g	g	g	g

Total

MEAL 2	CALORIES	CARBS	PROTEIN	FAT	SODIUM
	g	g	g	g	g
Time	g	g	g	g	g
:	g	g	g	g	g
	g	g	g	g	g

Total

MEAL 3	CALORIES	CARBS	PROTEIN	FAT	SODIUM
	g	g	g	g	g
Time	g	g	g	g	g
:	g	g	g	g	g
	g	g	g	g	g

Total

MEAL 4	CALORIES	CARBS	PROTEIN	FAT	SODIUM
	g	g	g	g	g
Time	g	g	g	g	g
:	g	g	g	g	g
	g	g	g	g	g

Total

MEAL 5	CALORIES	CARBS	PROTEIN	FAT	SODIUM
	g	g	g	g	g
Time	g	g	g	g	g
:	g	g	g	g	g
	g	g	g	g	g

Total

Tuesday _____   Month___   YR___

MEAL 1	CALORIES	CARBS	PROTEIN	FAT	SODIUM
	g	g	g	g	g
Time	g	g	g	g	g
:	g	g	g	g	g
	g	g	g	g	g

Total

MEAL 2	CALORIES	CARBS	PROTEIN	FAT	SODIUM
	g	g	g	g	g
Time	g	g	g	g	g
:	g	g	g	g	g
	g	g	g	g	g

Total

MEAL 3	CALORIES	CARBS	PROTEIN	FAT	SODIUM
	g	g	g	g	g
Time	g	g	g	g	g
:	g	g	g	g	g
	g	g	g	g	g

Total

MEAL 4	CALORIES	CARBS	PROTEIN	FAT	SODIUM
	g	g	g	g	g
Time	g	g	g	g	g
:	g	g	g	g	g
	g	g	g	g	g

Total

MEAL 5	CALORIES	CARBS	PROTEIN	FAT	SODIUM
	g	g	g	g	g
Time	g	g	g	g	g
:	g	g	g	g	g
	g	g	g	g	g

Total

Wednesday _____   Month___   YR___

MEAL 1 <u>CALORIES</u> <u>CARBS</u> <u>PROTEIN</u> <u>FAT</u> <u>SODIUM</u>
	g	g	g	g	g
Time	g	g	g	g	g
:	g	g	g	g	g
	g	g	g	g	g

Total

MEAL 2 <u>CALORIES</u> <u>CARBS</u> <u>PROTEIN</u> <u>FAT</u> <u>SODIUM</u>
	g	g	g	g	g
Time	g	g	g	g	g
:	g	g	g	g	g
	g	g	g	g	g

Total

MEAL 3 <u>CALORIES</u> <u>CARBS</u> <u>PROTEIN</u> <u>FAT</u> <u>SODIUM</u>
	g	g	g	g	g
Time	g	g	g	g	g
:	g	g	g	g	g
	g	g	g	g	g

Total

MEAL 4 <u>CALORIES</u> <u>CARBS</u> <u>PROTEIN</u> <u>FAT</u> <u>SODIUM</u>
	g	g	g	g	g
Time	g	g	g	g	g
:	g	g	g	g	g
	g	g	g	g	g

Total

MEAL 5 <u>CALORIES</u> <u>CARBS</u> <u>PROTEIN</u> <u>FAT</u> <u>SODIUM</u>
	g	g	g	g	g
Time	g	g	g	g	g
:	g	g	g	g	g
	g	g	g	g	g

Total

Thursday _____   Month___   YR___

MEAL 1 <u>CALORIES</u>   <u>CARBS</u>   <u>PROTEIN</u>   <u>FAT</u>   <u>SODIUM</u>

	CALORIES	CARBS	PROTEIN	FAT	SODIUM
	g	g	g	g	g
Time	g	g	g	g	g
:	g	g	g	g	g
	g	g	g	g	g

Total

MEAL 2 <u>CALORIES</u>   <u>CARBS</u>   <u>PROTEIN</u>   <u>FAT</u>   <u>SODIUM</u>

	CALORIES	CARBS	PROTEIN	FAT	SODIUM
	g	g	g	g	g
Time	g	g	g	g	g
:	g	g	g	g	g
	g	g	g	g	g

Total

MEAL 3 <u>CALORIES</u>   <u>CARBS</u>   <u>PROTEIN</u>   <u>FAT</u>   <u>SODIUM</u>

	CALORIES	CARBS	PROTEIN	FAT	SODIUM
	g	g	g	g	g
Time	g	g	g	g	g
:	g	g	g	g	g
	g	g	g	g	g

Total

MEAL 4 <u>CALORIES</u>   <u>CARBS</u>   <u>PROTEIN</u>   <u>FAT</u>   <u>SODIUM</u>

	CALORIES	CARBS	PROTEIN	FAT	SODIUM
	g	g	g	g	g
Time	g	g	g	g	g
:	g	g	g	g	g
	g	g	g	g	g

Total

MEAL 5 <u>CALORIES</u>   <u>CARBS</u>   <u>PROTEIN</u>   <u>FAT</u>   <u>SODIUM</u>

	CALORIES	CARBS	PROTEIN	FAT	SODIUM
	g	g	g	g	g
Time	g	g	g	g	g
:	g	g	g	g	g
	g	g	g	g	g

Total

Friday _____   Month___   YR___

MEAL 1	CALORIES	CARBS	PROTEIN	FAT	SODIUM
	g	g	g	g	g
Time	g	g	g	g	g
:	g	g	g	g	g
	g	g	g	g	g

Total

MEAL 2	CALORIES	CARBS	PROTEIN	FAT	SODIUM
	g	g	g	g	g
Time	g	g	g	g	g
:	g	g	g	g	g
	g	g	g	g	g

Total

MEAL 3	CALORIES	CARBS	PROTEIN	FAT	SODIUM
	g	g	g	g	g
Time	g	g	g	g	g
:	g	g	g	g	g
	g	g	g	g	g

Total

MEAL 4	CALORIES	CARBS	PROTEIN	FAT	SODIUM
	g	g	g	g	g
Time	g	g	g	g	g
:	g	g	g	g	g
	g	g	g	g	g

Total

MEAL 5	CALORIES	CARBS	PROTEIN	FAT	SODIUM
	g	g	g	g	g
Time	g	g	g	g	g
:	g	g	g	g	g
	g	g	g	g	g

Total

Saturday _____   Month___   YR___

MEAL 1 <u>CALORIES</u> <u>CARBS</u> <u>PROTEIN</u> <u>FAT</u> <u>SODIUM</u>

	g	g	g	g	g
Time	g	g	g	g	g
:	g	g	g	g	g
	g	g	g	g	g

Total

MEAL 2 <u>CALORIES</u> <u>CARBS</u> <u>PROTEIN</u> <u>FAT</u> <u>SODIUM</u>

	g	g	g	g	g
Time	g	g	g	g	g
:	g	g	g	g	g
	g	g	g	g	g

Total

MEAL 3 <u>CALORIES</u> <u>CARBS</u> <u>PROTEIN</u> <u>FAT</u> <u>SODIUM</u>

	g	g	g	g	g
Time	g	g	g	g	g
:	g	g	g	g	g
	g	g	g	g	g

Total

MEAL 4 <u>CALORIES</u> <u>CARBS</u> <u>PROTEIN</u> <u>FAT</u> <u>SODIUM</u>

	g	g	g	g	g
Time	g	g	g	g	g
:	g	g	g	g	g
	g	g	g	g	g

Total

MEAL 5 <u>CALORIES</u> <u>CARBS</u> <u>PROTEIN</u> <u>FAT</u> <u>SODIUM</u>

	g	g	g	g	g
Time	g	g	g	g	g
:	g	g	g	g	g
	g	g	g	g	g

Total

Notes

Sunday _____   Month____   YR___

MEAL 1	CALORIES	CARBS	PROTEIN	FAT	SODIUM
	g	g	g	g	g
Time	g	g	g	g	g
:	g	g	g	g	g
	g	g	g	g	g

Total

MEAL 2	CALORIES	CARBS	PROTEIN	FAT	SODIUM
	g	g	g	g	g
Time	g	g	g	g	g
:	g	g	g	g	g
	g	g	g	g	g

Total

MEAL 3	CALORIES	CARBS	PROTEIN	FAT	SODIUM
	g	g	g	g	g
Time	g	g	g	g	g
:	g	g	g	g	g
	g	g	g	g	g

Total

MEAL 4	CALORIES	CARBS	PROTEIN	FAT	SODIUM
	g	g	g	g	g
Time	g	g	g	g	g
:	g	g	g	g	g
	g	g	g	g	g

Total

MEAL 5	CALORIES	CARBS	PROTEIN	FAT	SODIUM
	g	g	g	g	g
Time	g	g	g	g	g
:	g	g	g	g	g
	g	g	g	g	g

Total

Monday _____   Month___ YR___

MEAL 1	CALORIES	CARBS	PROTEIN	FAT	SODIUM
	g	g	g	g	g
Time	g	g	g	g	g
:	g	g	g	g	g
	g	g	g	g	g

Total

MEAL 2	CALORIES	CARBS	PROTEIN	FAT	SODIUM
	g	g	g	g	g
Time	g	g	g	g	g
:	g	g	g	g	g
	g	g	g	g	g

Total

MEAL 3	CALORIES	CARBS	PROTEIN	FAT	SODIUM
	g	g	g	g	g
Time	g	g	g	g	g
:	g	g	g	g	g
	g	g	g	g	g

Total

MEAL 4	CALORIES	CARBS	PROTEIN	FAT	SODIUM
	g	g	g	g	g
Time	g	g	g	g	g
:	g	g	g	g	g
	g	g	g	g	g

Total

MEAL 5	CALORIES	CARBS	PROTEIN	FAT	SODIUM
	g	g	g	g	g
Time	g	g	g	g	g
:	g	g	g	g	g
	g	g	g	g	g

Total

Tuesday _____   Month____   YR___

MEAL 1	CALORIES	CARBS	PROTEIN	FAT	SODIUM
	g	g	g	g	g
Time	g	g	g	g	g
:	g	g	g	g	g
	g	g	g	g	g

Total

MEAL 2	CALORIES	CARBS	PROTEIN	FAT	SODIUM
	g	g	g	g	g
Time	g	g	g	g	g
:	g	g	g	g	g
	g	g	g	g	g

Total

MEAL 3	CALORIES	CARBS	PROTEIN	FAT	SODIUM
	g	g	g	g	g
Time	g	g	g	g	g
:	g	g	g	g	g
	g	g	g	g	g

Total

MEAL 4	CALORIES	CARBS	PROTEIN	FAT	SODIUM
	g	g	g	g	g
Time	g	g	g	g	g
:	g	g	g	g	g
	g	g	g	g	g

Total

MEAL 5	CALORIES	CARBS	PROTEIN	FAT	SODIUM
	g	g	g	g	g
Time	g	g	g	g	g
:	g	g	g	g	g
	g	g	g	g	g

Total

Wednesday_____   Month___   YR___

MEAL 1	CALORIES	CARBS	PROTEIN	FAT	SODIUM
	g	g	g	g	g
Time	g	g	g	g	g
:	g	g	g	g	g
	g	g	g	g	g

Total

MEAL 2	CALORIES	CARBS	PROTEIN	FAT	SODIUM
	g	g	g	g	g
Time	g	g	g	g	g
:	g	g	g	g	g
	g	g	g	g	g

Total

MEAL 3	CALORIES	CARBS	PROTEIN	FAT	SODIUM
	g	g	g	g	g
Time	g	g	g	g	g
:	g	g	g	g	g
	g	g	g	g	g

Total

MEAL 4	CALORIES	CARBS	PROTEIN	FAT	SODIUM
	g	g	g	g	g
Time	g	g	g	g	g
:	g	g	g	g	g
	g	g	g	g	g

Total

MEAL 5	CALORIES	CARBS	PROTEIN	FAT	SODIUM
	g	g	g	g	g
Time	g	g	g	g	g
:	g	g	g	g	g
	g	g	g	g	g

Total

Thursday _____   Month___   YR___

MEAL 1 <u>CALORIES</u> <u>CARBS</u>   <u>PROTEIN</u>   <u>FAT</u>   <u>SODIUM</u>
	g	g	g	g	g
Time	g	g	g	g	g
:	g	g	g	g	g
	g	g	g	g	g

Total

MEAL 2 <u>CALORIES</u> <u>CARBS</u>   <u>PROTEIN</u>   <u>FAT</u>   <u>SODIUM</u>
	g	g	g	g	g
Time	g	g	g	g	g
:	g	g	g	g	g
	g	g	g	g	g

Total

MEAL 3 <u>CALORIES</u> <u>CARBS</u>   <u>PROTEIN</u>   <u>FAT</u>   <u>SODIUM</u>
	g	g	g	g	g
Time	g	g	g	g	g
:	g	g	g	g	g
	g	g	g	g	g

Total

MEAL 4 <u>CALORIES</u> <u>CARBS</u>   <u>PROTEIN</u>   <u>FAT</u>   <u>SODIUM</u>
	g	g	g	g	g
Time	g	g	g	g	g
:	g	g	g	g	g
	g	g	g	g	g

Total

MEAL 5 <u>CALORIES</u> <u>CARBS</u>   <u>PROTEIN</u>   <u>FAT</u>   <u>SODIUM</u>
	g	g	g	g	g
Time	g	g	g	g	g
:	g	g	g	g	g
	g	g	g	g	g

Total

Friday _____   Month___   YR___

MEAL 1	CALORIES	CARBS	PROTEIN	FAT	SODIUM
	g	g	g	g	g
Time	g	g	g	g	g
:	g	g	g	g	g
	g	g	g	g	g

Total

MEAL 2	CALORIES	CARBS	PROTEIN	FAT	SODIUM
	g	g	g	g	g
Time	g	g	g	g	g
:	g	g	g	g	g
	g	g	g	g	g

Total

MEAL 3	CALORIES	CARBS	PROTEIN	FAT	SODIUM
	g	g	g	g	g
Time	g	g	g	g	g
:	g	g	g	g	g
	g	g	g	g	g

Total

MEAL 4	CALORIES	CARBS	PROTEIN	FAT	SODIUM
	g	g	g	g	g
Time	g	g	g	g	g
:	g	g	g	g	g
	g	g	g	g	g

Total

MEAL 5	CALORIES	CARBS	PROTEIN	FAT	SODIUM
	g	g	g	g	g
Time	g	g	g	g	g
:	g	g	g	g	g
	g	g	g	g	g

Total

Saturday _____   Month___   YR___

MEAL 1	CALORIES	CARBS	PROTEIN	FAT	SODIUM
	g	g	g	g	g
Time	g	g	g	g	g
:	g	g	g	g	g
	g	g	g	g	g

Total

MEAL 2	CALORIES	CARBS	PROTEIN	FAT	SODIUM
	g	g	g	g	g
Time	g	g	g	g	g
:	g	g	g	g	g
	g	g	g	g	g

Total

MEAL 3	CALORIES	CARBS	PROTEIN	FAT	SODIUM
	g	g	g	g	g
Time	g	g	g	g	g
:	g	g	g	g	g
	g	g	g	g	g

Total

MEAL 4	CALORIES	CARBS	PROTEIN	FAT	SODIUM
	g	g	g	g	g
Time	g	g	g	g	g
:	g	g	g	g	g
	g	g	g	g	g

Total

MEAL 5	CALORIES	CARBS	PROTEIN	FAT	SODIUM
	g	g	g	g	g
Time	g	g	g	g	g
:	g	g	g	g	g
	g	g	g	g	g

Total

Notes

Sunday _____   Month___   YR___

MEAL 1	CALORIES	CARBS	PROTEIN	FAT	SODIUM
	g	g	g	g	g
Time	g	g	g	g	g
:	g	g	g	g	g
	g	g	g	g	g

Total

MEAL 2	CALORIES	CARBS	PROTEIN	FAT	SODIUM
	g	g	g	g	g
Time	g	g	g	g	g
:	g	g	g	g	g
	g	g	g	g	g

Total

MEAL 3	CALORIES	CARBS	PROTEIN	FAT	SODIUM
	g	g	g	g	g
Time	g	g	g	g	g
:	g	g	g	g	g
	g	g	g	g	g

Total

MEAL 4	CALORIES	CARBS	PROTEIN	FAT	SODIUM
	g	g	g	g	g
Time	g	g	g	g	g
:	g	g	g	g	g
	g	g	g	g	g

Total

MEAL 5	CALORIES	CARBS	PROTEIN	FAT	SODIUM
	g	g	g	g	g
Time	g	g	g	g	g
:	g	g	g	g	g
	g	g	g	g	g

Total

Monday _____   Month___   YR___

MEAL 1	CALORIES	CARBS	PROTEIN	FAT	SODIUM
	g	g	g	g	g
Time	g	g	g	g	g
:	g	g	g	g	g
	g	g	g	g	g

Total

MEAL 2	CALORIES	CARBS	PROTEIN	FAT	SODIUM
	g	g	g	g	g
Time	g	g	g	g	g
:	g	g	g	g	g
	g	g	g	g	g

Total

MEAL 3	CALORIES	CARBS	PROTEIN	FAT	SODIUM
	g	g	g	g	g
Time	g	g	g	g	g
:	g	g	g	g	g
	g	g	g	g	g

Total

MEAL 4	CALORIES	CARBS	PROTEIN	FAT	SODIUM
	g	g	g	g	g
Time	g	g	g	g	g
:	g	g	g	g	g
	g	g	g	g	g

Total

MEAL 5	CALORIES	CARBS	PROTEIN	FAT	SODIUM
	g	g	g	g	g
Time	g	g	g	g	g
:	g	g	g	g	g
	g	g	g	g	g

Total

Tuesday _____   Month____ YR____

MEAL 1	CALORIES	CARBS	PROTEIN	FAT	SODIUM
	g	g	g	g	g
Time	g	g	g	g	g
:	g	g	g	g	g
	g	g	g	g	g

Total

MEAL 2	CALORIES	CARBS	PROTEIN	FAT	SODIUM
	g	g	g	g	g
Time	g	g	g	g	g
:	g	g	g	g	g
	g	g	g	g	g

Total

MEAL 3	CALORIES	CARBS	PROTEIN	FAT	SODIUM
	g	g	g	g	g
Time	g	g	g	g	g
:	g	g	g	g	g
	g	g	g	g	g

Total

MEAL 4	CALORIES	CARBS	PROTEIN	FAT	SODIUM
	g	g	g	g	g
Time	g	g	g	g	g
:	g	g	g	g	g
	g	g	g	g	g

Total

MEAL 5	CALORIES	CARBS	PROTEIN	FAT	SODIUM
	g	g	g	g	g
Time	g	g	g	g	g
:	g	g	g	g	g
	g	g	g	g	g

Total

Wednesday _____   Month___ YR___

MEAL 1 <u>CALORIES</u> <u>CARBS</u> <u>PROTEIN</u> <u>FAT</u> <u>SODIUM</u>

	g	g	g	g	g
Time	g	g	g	g	g
:	g	g	g	g	g
	g	g	g	g	g

Total

MEAL 2 <u>CALORIES</u> <u>CARBS</u> <u>PROTEIN</u> <u>FAT</u> <u>SODIUM</u>

	g	g	g	g	g
Time	g	g	g	g	g
:	g	g	g	g	g
	g	g	g	g	g

Total

MEAL 3 <u>CALORIES</u> <u>CARBS</u> <u>PROTEIN</u> <u>FAT</u> <u>SODIUM</u>

	g	g	g	g	g
Time	g	g	g	g	g
:	g	g	g	g	g
	g	g	g	g	g

Total

MEAL 4 <u>CALORIES</u> <u>CARBS</u> <u>PROTEIN</u> <u>FAT</u> <u>SODIUM</u>

	g	g	g	g	g
Time	g	g	g	g	g
:	g	g	g	g	g
	g	g	g	g	g

Total

MEAL 5 <u>CALORIES</u> <u>CARBS</u> <u>PROTEIN</u> <u>FAT</u> <u>SODIUM</u>

	g	g	g	g	g
Time	g	g	g	g	g
:	g	g	g	g	g
	g	g	g	g	g

Total

Thursday _____   Month___   YR___

MEAL 1	CALORIES	CARBS	PROTEIN	FAT	SODIUM
	g	g	g	g	g
Time	g	g	g	g	g
:	g	g	g	g	g
	g	g	g	g	g

Total

MEAL 2	CALORIES	CARBS	PROTEIN	FAT	SODIUM
	g	g	g	g	g
Time	g	g	g	g	g
:	g	g	g	g	g
	g	g	g	g	g

Total

MEAL 3	CALORIES	CARBS	PROTEIN	FAT	SODIUM
	g	g	g	g	g
Time	g	g	g	g	g
:	g	g	g	g	g
	g	g	g	g	g

Total

MEAL 4	CALORIES	CARBS	PROTEIN	FAT	SODIUM
	g	g	g	g	g
Time	g	g	g	g	g
:	g	g	g	g	g
	g	g	g	g	g

Total

MEAL 5	CALORIES	CARBS	PROTEIN	FAT	SODIUM
	g	g	g	g	g
Time	g	g	g	g	g
:	g	g	g	g	g
	g	g	g	g	g

Total

Friday _____   Month___   YR___

MEAL 1 <u>CALORIES</u>   <u>CARBS</u>   <u>PROTEIN</u>   <u>FAT</u>   <u>SODIUM</u>
	g	g	g	g	g
Time	g	g	g	g	g
:	g	g	g	g	g
	g	g	g	g	g

Total

MEAL 2 <u>CALORIES</u>   <u>CARBS</u>   <u>PROTEIN</u>   <u>FAT</u>   <u>SODIUM</u>
	g	g	g	g	g
Time	g	g	g	g	g
:	g	g	g	g	g
	g	g	g	g	g

Total

MEAL 3 <u>CALORIES</u>   <u>CARBS</u>   <u>PROTEIN</u>   <u>FAT</u>   <u>SODIUM</u>
	g	g	g	g	g
Time	g	g	g	g	g
:	g	g	g	g	g
	g	g	g	g	g

Total

MEAL 4 <u>CALORIES</u>   <u>CARBS</u>   <u>PROTEIN</u>   <u>FAT</u>   <u>SODIUM</u>
	g	g	g	g	g
Time	g	g	g	g	g
:	g	g	g	g	g
	g	g	g	g	g

Total

MEAL 5 <u>CALORIES</u>   <u>CARBS</u>   <u>PROTEIN</u>   <u>FAT</u>   <u>SODIUM</u>
	g	g	g	g	g
Time	g	g	g	g	g
:	g	g	g	g	g
	g	g	g	g	g

Total

Saturday _____   Month___   YR___

MEAL 1	<u>CALORIES</u>	<u>CARBS</u>	<u>PROTEIN</u>	<u>FAT</u>	<u>SODIUM</u>
	g	g	g	g	g
Time	g	g	g	g	g
:	g	g	g	g	g
	g	g	g	g	g

Total

MEAL 2	<u>CALORIES</u>	<u>CARBS</u>	<u>PROTEIN</u>	<u>FAT</u>	<u>SODIUM</u>
	g	g	g	g	g
Time	g	g	g	g	g
:	g	g	g	g	g
	g	g	g	g	g

Total

MEAL 3	<u>CALORIES</u>	<u>CARBS</u>	<u>PROTEIN</u>	<u>FAT</u>	<u>SODIUM</u>
	g	g	g	g	g
Time	g	g	g	g	g
:	g	g	g	g	g
	g	g	g	g	g

Total

MEAL 4	<u>CALORIES</u>	<u>CARBS</u>	<u>PROTEIN</u>	<u>FAT</u>	<u>SODIUM</u>
	g	g	g	g	g
Time	g	g	g	g	g
:	g	g	g	g	g
	g	g	g	g	g

Total

MEAL 5	<u>CALORIES</u>	<u>CARBS</u>	<u>PROTEIN</u>	<u>FAT</u>	<u>SODIUM</u>
	g	g	g	g	g
Time	g	g	g	g	g
:	g	g	g	g	g
	g	g	g	g	g

Total

Notes

_____

_____

_____

_____

_____

_____

_____

_____

_____

_____

_____

_____

_____

_____

_____

_____

_____

_____

Sunday _____   Month____   YR____

MEAL 1	CALORIES	CARBS	PROTEIN	FAT	SODIUM
	g	g	g	g	g
Time	g	g	g	g	g
:	g	g	g	g	g
	g	g	g	g	g

Total

MEAL 2	CALORIES	CARBS	PROTEIN	FAT	SODIUM
	g	g	g	g	g
Time	g	g	g	g	g
:	g	g	g	g	g
	g	g	g	g	g

Total

MEAL 3	CALORIES	CARBS	PROTEIN	FAT	SODIUM
	g	g	g	g	g
Time	g	g	g	g	g
:	g	g	g	g	g
	g	g	g	g	g

Total

MEAL 4	CALORIES	CARBS	PROTEIN	FAT	SODIUM
	g	g	g	g	g
Time	g	g	g	g	g
:	g	g	g	g	g
	g	g	g	g	g

Total

MEAL 5	CALORIES	CARBS	PROTEIN	FAT	SODIUM
	g	g	g	g	g
Time	g	g	g	g	g
:	g	g	g	g	g
	g	g	g	g	g

Total

Monday _____   Month___   YR___

MEAL 1	CALORIES	CARBS	PROTEIN	FAT	SODIUM
	g	g	g	g	g
Time	g	g	g	g	g
:	g	g	g	g	g
	g	g	g	g	g

Total

MEAL 2	CALORIES	CARBS	PROTEIN	FAT	SODIUM
	g	g	g	g	g
Time	g	g	g	g	g
:	g	g	g	g	g
	g	g	g	g	g

Total

MEAL 3	CALORIES	CARBS	PROTEIN	FAT	SODIUM
	g	g	g	g	g
Time	g	g	g	g	g
:	g	g	g	g	g
	g	g	g	g	g

Total

MEAL 4	CALORIES	CARBS	PROTEIN	FAT	SODIUM
	g	g	g	g	g
Time	g	g	g	g	g
:	g	g	g	g	g
	g	g	g	g	g

Total

MEAL 5	CALORIES	CARBS	PROTEIN	FAT	SODIUM
	g	g	g	g	g
Time	g	g	g	g	g
:	g	g	g	g	g
	g	g	g	g	g

Total

Tuesday _____   Month___   YR___

MEAL 1	CALORIES	CARBS	PROTEIN	FAT	SODIUM
	g	g	g	g	g
Time	g	g	g	g	g
:	g	g	g	g	g
	g	g	g	g	g

Total

MEAL 2	CALORIES	CARBS	PROTEIN	FAT	SODIUM
	g	g	g	g	g
Time	g	g	g	g	g
:	g	g	g	g	g
	g	g	g	g	g

Total

MEAL 3	CALORIES	CARBS	PROTEIN	FAT	SODIUM
	g	g	g	g	g
Time	g	g	g	g	g
:	g	g	g	g	g
	g	g	g	g	g

Total

MEAL 4	CALORIES	CARBS	PROTEIN	FAT	SODIUM
	g	g	g	g	g
Time	g	g	g	g	g
:	g	g	g	g	g
	g	g	g	g	g

Total

MEAL 5	CALORIES	CARBS	PROTEIN	FAT	SODIUM
	g	g	g	g	g
Time	g	g	g	g	g
:	g	g	g	g	g
	g	g	g	g	g

Total

Wednesday _____   Month___   YR___

MEAL 1	CALORIES	CARBS	PROTEIN	FAT	SODIUM
	g	g	g	g	g
Time	g	g	g	g	g
:	g	g	g	g	g
	g	g	g	g	g

Total

MEAL 2	CALORIES	CARBS	PROTEIN	FAT	SODIUM
	g	g	g	g	g
Time	g	g	g	g	g
:	g	g	g	g	g
	g	g	g	g	g

Total

MEAL 3	CALORIES	CARBS	PROTEIN	FAT	SODIUM
	g	g	g	g	g
Time	g	g	g	g	g
:	g	g	g	g	g
	g	g	g	g	g

Total

MEAL 4	CALORIES	CARBS	PROTEIN	FAT	SODIUM
	g	g	g	g	g
Time	g	g	g	g	g
:	g	g	g	g	g
	g	g	g	g	g

Total

MEAL 5	CALORIES	CARBS	PROTEIN	FAT	SODIUM
	g	g	g	g	g
Time	g	g	g	g	g
:	g	g	g	g	g
	g	g	g	g	g

Total

Thursday _____   Month___   YR___

MEAL 1	CALORIES	CARBS	PROTEIN	FAT	SODIUM
	g	g	g	g	g
Time	g	g	g	g	g
:	g	g	g	g	g
	g	g	g	g	g

Total

MEAL 2	CALORIES	CARBS	PROTEIN	FAT	SODIUM
	g	g	g	g	g
Time	g	g	g	g	g
:	g	g	g	g	g
	g	g	g	g	g

Total

MEAL 3	CALORIES	CARBS	PROTEIN	FAT	SODIUM
	g	g	g	g	g
Time	g	g	g	g	g
:	g	g	g	g	g
	g	g	g	g	g

Total

MEAL 4	CALORIES	CARBS	PROTEIN	FAT	SODIUM
	g	g	g	g	g
Time	g	g	g	g	g
:	g	g	g	g	g
	g	g	g	g	g

Total

MEAL 5	CALORIES	CARBS	PROTEIN	FAT	SODIUM
	g	g	g	g	g
Time	g	g	g	g	g
:	g	g	g	g	g
	g	g	g	g	g

Total

Friday _____   Month___   YR___

MEAL 1	CALORIES	CARBS	PROTEIN	FAT	SODIUM
	g	g	g	g	g
Time	g	g	g	g	g
:	g	g	g	g	g
	g	g	g	g	g

Total

MEAL 2	CALORIES	CARBS	PROTEIN	FAT	SODIUM
	g	g	g	g	g
Time	g	g	g	g	g
:	g	g	g	g	g
	g	g	g	g	g

Total

MEAL 3	CALORIES	CARBS	PROTEIN	FAT	SODIUM
	g	g	g	g	g
Time	g	g	g	g	g
:	g	g	g	g	g
	g	g	g	g	g

Total

MEAL 4	CALORIES	CARBS	PROTEIN	FAT	SODIUM
	g	g	g	g	g
Time	g	g	g	g	g
:	g	g	g	g	g
	g	g	g	g	g

Total

MEAL 5	CALORIES	CARBS	PROTEIN	FAT	SODIUM
	g	g	g	g	g
Time	g	g	g	g	g
:	g	g	g	g	g
	g	g	g	g	g

Total

Saturday _____   Month___   YR___

MEAL 1	CALORIES	CARBS	PROTEIN	FAT	SODIUM
	g	g	g	g	g
Time	g	g	g	g	g
:	g	g	g	g	g
	g	g	g	g	g

Total

MEAL 2	CALORIES	CARBS	PROTEIN	FAT	SODIUM
	g	g	g	g	g
Time	g	g	g	g	g
:	g	g	g	g	g
	g	g	g	g	g

Total

MEAL 3	CALORIES	CARBS	PROTEIN	FAT	SODIUM
	g	g	g	g	g
Time	g	g	g	g	g
:	g	g	g	g	g
	g	g	g	g	g

Total

MEAL 4	CALORIES	CARBS	PROTEIN	FAT	SODIUM
	g	g	g	g	g
Time	g	g	g	g	g
:	g	g	g	g	g
	g	g	g	g	g

Total

MEAL 5	CALORIES	CARBS	PROTEIN	FAT	SODIUM
	g	g	g	g	g
Time	g	g	g	g	g
:	g	g	g	g	g
	g	g	g	g	g

Total

Notes

_____

_____

_____

_____

_____

_____

_____

_____

_____

_____

_____

_____

_____

_____

_____

_____

_____

Sunday _____   Month___   YR___

MEAL 1	CALORIES	CARBS	PROTEIN	FAT	SODIUM
	g	g	g	g	g
Time	g	g	g	g	g
:	g	g	g	g	g
	g	g	g	g	g

Total

MEAL 2	CALORIES	CARBS	PROTEIN	FAT	SODIUM
	g	g	g	g	g
Time	g	g	g	g	g
:	g	g	g	g	g
	g	g	g	g	g

Total

MEAL 3	CALORIES	CARBS	PROTEIN	FAT	SODIUM
	g	g	g	g	g
Time	g	g	g	g	g
:	g	g	g	g	g
	g	g	g	g	g

Total

MEAL 4	CALORIES	CARBS	PROTEIN	FAT	SODIUM
	g	g	g	g	g
Time	g	g	g	g	g
:	g	g	g	g	g
	g	g	g	g	g

Total

MEAL 5	CALORIES	CARBS	PROTEIN	FAT	SODIUM
	g	g	g	g	g
Time	g	g	g	g	g
:	g	g	g	g	g
	g	g	g	g	g

Total

Monday _____   Month___   YR___

MEAL 1	CALORIES	CARBS	PROTEIN	FAT	SODIUM
	g	g	g	g	g
Time	g	g	g	g	g
:	g	g	g	g	g
	g	g	g	g	g

Total

MEAL 2	CALORIES	CARBS	PROTEIN	FAT	SODIUM
	g	g	g	g	g
Time	g	g	g	g	g
:	g	g	g	g	g
	g	g	g	g	g

Total

MEAL 3	CALORIES	CARBS	PROTEIN	FAT	SODIUM
	g	g	g	g	g
Time	g	g	g	g	g
:	g	g	g	g	g
	g	g	g	g	g

Total

MEAL 4	CALORIES	CARBS	PROTEIN	FAT	SODIUM
	g	g	g	g	g
Time	g	g	g	g	g
:	g	g	g	g	g
	g	g	g	g	g

Total

MEAL 5	CALORIES	CARBS	PROTEIN	FAT	SODIUM
	g	g	g	g	g
Time	g	g	g	g	g
:	g	g	g	g	g
	g	g	g	g	g

Total

Tuesday _____   Month___   YR___

MEAL 1 <u>CALORIES</u>   <u>CARBS</u>   <u>PROTEIN</u>   <u>FAT</u>   <u>SODIUM</u>

	CALORIES	CARBS	PROTEIN	FAT	SODIUM
	g	g	g	g	g
Time	g	g	g	g	g
:	g	g	g	g	g
	g	g	g	g	g

Total

MEAL 2 <u>CALORIES</u>   <u>CARBS</u>   <u>PROTEIN</u>   <u>FAT</u>   <u>SODIUM</u>

	CALORIES	CARBS	PROTEIN	FAT	SODIUM
	g	g	g	g	g
Time	g	g	g	g	g
:	g	g	g	g	g
	g	g	g	g	g

Total

MEAL 3 <u>CALORIES</u>   <u>CARBS</u>   <u>PROTEIN</u>   <u>FAT</u>   <u>SODIUM</u>

	CALORIES	CARBS	PROTEIN	FAT	SODIUM
	g	g	g	g	g
Time	g	g	g	g	g
:	g	g	g	g	g
	g	g	g	g	g

Total

MEAL 4 <u>CALORIES</u>   <u>CARBS</u>   <u>PROTEIN</u>   <u>FAT</u>   <u>SODIUM</u>

	CALORIES	CARBS	PROTEIN	FAT	SODIUM
	g	g	g	g	g
Time	g	g	g	g	g
:	g	g	g	g	g
	g	g	g	g	g

Total

MEAL 5 <u>CALORIES</u>   <u>CARBS</u>   <u>PROTEIN</u>   <u>FAT</u>   <u>SODIUM</u>

	CALORIES	CARBS	PROTEIN	FAT	SODIUM
	g	g	g	g	g
Time	g	g	g	g	g
:	g	g	g	g	g
	g	g	g	g	g

Total

Wednesday _____   Month___   YR___

MEAL 1	CALORIES	CARBS	PROTEIN	FAT	SODIUM
	g	g	g	g	g
Time	g	g	g	g	g
:	g	g	g	g	g
	g	g	g	g	g

Total

MEAL 2	CALORIES	CARBS	PROTEIN	FAT	SODIUM
	g	g	g	g	g
Time	g	g	g	g	g
:	g	g	g	g	g
	g	g	g	g	g

Total

MEAL 3	CALORIES	CARBS	PROTEIN	FAT	SODIUM
	g	g	g	g	g
Time	g	g	g	g	g
:	g	g	g	g	g
	g	g	g	g	g

Total

MEAL 4	CALORIES	CARBS	PROTEIN	FAT	SODIUM
	g	g	g	g	g
Time	g	g	g	g	g
:	g	g	g	g	g
	g	g	g	g	g

Total

MEAL 5	CALORIES	CARBS	PROTEIN	FAT	SODIUM
	g	g	g	g	g
Time	g	g	g	g	g
:	g	g	g	g	g
	g	g	g	g	g

Total

Thursday _____   Month___   YR___

MEAL 1	CALORIES	CARBS	PROTEIN	FAT	SODIUM
	g	g	g	g	g
Time	g	g	g	g	g
:	g	g	g	g	g
	g	g	g	g	g

Total

MEAL 2	CALORIES	CARBS	PROTEIN	FAT	SODIUM
	g	g	g	g	g
Time	g	g	g	g	g
:	g	g	g	g	g
	g	g	g	g	g

Total

MEAL 3	CALORIES	CARBS	PROTEIN	FAT	SODIUM
	g	g	g	g	g
Time	g	g	g	g	g
:	g	g	g	g	g
	g	g	g	g	g

Total

MEAL 4	CALORIES	CARBS	PROTEIN	FAT	SODIUM
	g	g	g	g	g
Time	g	g	g	g	g
:	g	g	g	g	g
	g	g	g	g	g

Total

MEAL 5	CALORIES	CARBS	PROTEIN	FAT	SODIUM
	g	g	g	g	g
Time	g	g	g	g	g
:	g	g	g	g	g
	g	g	g	g	g

Total

Friday _____   Month___   YR___

MEAL 1	CALORIES	CARBS	PROTEIN	FAT	SODIUM
	g	g	g	g	g
Time	g	g	g	g	g
:	g	g	g	g	g
	g	g	g	g	g

Total

MEAL 2	CALORIES	CARBS	PROTEIN	FAT	SODIUM
	g	g	g	g	g
Time	g	g	g	g	g
:	g	g	g	g	g
	g	g	g	g	g

Total

MEAL 3	CALORIES	CARBS	PROTEIN	FAT	SODIUM
	g	g	g	g	g
Time	g	g	g	g	g
:	g	g	g	g	g
	g	g	g	g	g

Total

MEAL 4	CALORIES	CARBS	PROTEIN	FAT	SODIUM
	g	g	g	g	g
Time	g	g	g	g	g
:	g	g	g	g	g
	g	g	g	g	g

Total

MEAL 5	CALORIES	CARBS	PROTEIN	FAT	SODIUM
	g	g	g	g	g
Time	g	g	g	g	g
:	g	g	g	g	g
	g	g	g	g	g

Total

Saturday _____   Month___   YR___

MEAL 1	CALORIES	CARBS	PROTEIN	FAT	SODIUM
	g	g	g	g	g
Time	g	g	g	g	g
:	g	g	g	g	g
	g	g	g	g	g

Total

MEAL 2	CALORIES	CARBS	PROTEIN	FAT	SODIUM
	g	g	g	g	g
Time	g	g	g	g	g
:	g	g	g	g	g
	g	g	g	g	g

Total

MEAL 3	CALORIES	CARBS	PROTEIN	FAT	SODIUM
	g	g	g	g	g
Time	g	g	g	g	g
:	g	g	g	g	g
	g	g	g	g	g

Total

MEAL 4	CALORIES	CARBS	PROTEIN	FAT	SODIUM
	g	g	g	g	g
Time	g	g	g	g	g
:	g	g	g	g	g
	g	g	g	g	g

Total

MEAL 5	CALORIES	CARBS	PROTEIN	FAT	SODIUM
	g	g	g	g	g
Time	g	g	g	g	g
:	g	g	g	g	g
	g	g	g	g	g

Total

Notes

Sunday_____   Month___   YR___

MEAL 1	CALORIES	CARBS	PROTEIN	FAT	SODIUM
	g	g	g	g	g
Time	g	g	g	g	g
:	g	g	g	g	g
	g	g	g	g	g

Total

MEAL 2	CALORIES	CARBS	PROTEIN	FAT	SODIUM
	g	g	g	g	g
Time	g	g	g	g	g
:	g	g	g	g	g
	g	g	g	g	g

Total

MEAL 3	CALORIES	CARBS	PROTEIN	FAT	SODIUM
	g	g	g	g	g
Time	g	g	g	g	g
:	g	g	g	g	g
	g	g	g	g	g

Total

MEAL 4	CALORIES	CARBS	PROTEIN	FAT	SODIUM
	g	g	g	g	g
Time	g	g	g	g	g
:	g	g	g	g	g
	g	g	g	g	g

Total

MEAL 5	CALORIES	CARBS	PROTEIN	FAT	SODIUM
	g	g	g	g	g
Time	g	g	g	g	g
:	g	g	g	g	g
	g	g	g	g	g

Total

Monday _____   Month___   YR___

MEAL 1	CALORIES	CARBS	PROTEIN	FAT	SODIUM
	g	g	g	g	g
Time	g	g	g	g	g
:	g	g	g	g	g
	g	g	g	g	g

Total

MEAL 2	CALORIES	CARBS	PROTEIN	FAT	SODIUM
	g	g	g	g	g
Time	g	g	g	g	g
:	g	g	g	g	g
	g	g	g	g	g

Total

MEAL 3	CALORIES	CARBS	PROTEIN	FAT	SODIUM
	g	g	g	g	g
Time	g	g	g	g	g
:	g	g	g	g	g
	g	g	g	g	g

Total

MEAL 4	CALORIES	CARBS	PROTEIN	FAT	SODIUM
	g	g	g	g	g
Time	g	g	g	g	g
:	g	g	g	g	g
	g	g	g	g	g

Total

MEAL 5	CALORIES	CARBS	PROTEIN	FAT	SODIUM
	g	g	g	g	g
Time	g	g	g	g	g
:	g	g	g	g	g
	g	g	g	g	g

Total

Tuesday _____   Month___   YR___

MEAL 1	CALORIES	CARBS	PROTEIN	FAT	SODIUM
	g	g	g	g	g
Time	g	g	g	g	g
:	g	g	g	g	g
	g	g	g	g	g

Total

MEAL 2	CALORIES	CARBS	PROTEIN	FAT	SODIUM
	g	g	g	g	g
Time	g	g	g	g	g
:	g	g	g	g	g
	g	g	g	g	g

Total

MEAL 3	CALORIES	CARBS	PROTEIN	FAT	SODIUM
	g	g	g	g	g
Time	g	g	g	g	g
:	g	g	g	g	g
	g	g	g	g	g

Total

MEAL 4	CALORIES	CARBS	PROTEIN	FAT	SODIUM
	g	g	g	g	g
Time	g	g	g	g	g
:	g	g	g	g	g
	g	g	g	g	g

Total

MEAL 5	CALORIES	CARBS	PROTEIN	FAT	SODIUM
	g	g	g	g	g
Time	g	g	g	g	g
:	g	g	g	g	g
	g	g	g	g	g

Total

Wednesday _____   Month___ YR___

MEAL 1 <u>CALORIES</u> <u>CARBS</u> <u>PROTEIN</u> <u>FAT</u> <u>SODIUM</u>
	g	g	g	g	g
Time	g	g	g	g	g
:	g	g	g	g	g
	g	g	g	g	g

Total

MEAL 2 <u>CALORIES</u> <u>CARBS</u> <u>PROTEIN</u> <u>FAT</u> <u>SODIUM</u>
	g	g	g	g	g
Time	g	g	g	g	g
:	g	g	g	g	g
	g	g	g	g	g

Total

MEAL 3 <u>CALORIES</u> <u>CARBS</u> <u>PROTEIN</u> <u>FAT</u> <u>SODIUM</u>
	g	g	g	g	g
Time	g	g	g	g	g
:	g	g	g	g	g
	g	g	g	g	g

Total

MEAL 4 <u>CALORIES</u> <u>CARBS</u> <u>PROTEIN</u> <u>FAT</u> <u>SODIUM</u>
	g	g	g	g	g
Time	g	g	g	g	g
:	g	g	g	g	g
	g	g	g	g	g

Total

MEAL 5 <u>CALORIES</u> <u>CARBS</u> <u>PROTEIN</u> <u>FAT</u> <u>SODIUM</u>
	g	g	g	g	g
Time	g	g	g	g	g
:	g	g	g	g	g
	g	g	g	g	g

Total

Thursday _____   Month___   YR___

MEAL 1	CALORIES	CARBS	PROTEIN	FAT	SODIUM
	g	g	g	g	g
Time	g	g	g	g	g
:	g	g	g	g	g
	g	g	g	g	g

Total

MEAL 2	CALORIES	CARBS	PROTEIN	FAT	SODIUM
	g	g	g	g	g
Time	g	g	g	g	g
:	g	g	g	g	g
	g	g	g	g	g

Total

MEAL 3	CALORIES	CARBS	PROTEIN	FAT	SODIUM
	g	g	g	g	g
Time	g	g	g	g	g
:	g	g	g	g	g
	g	g	g	g	g

Total

MEAL 4	CALORIES	CARBS	PROTEIN	FAT	SODIUM
	g	g	g	g	g
Time	g	g	g	g	g
:	g	g	g	g	g
	g	g	g	g	g

Total

MEAL 5	CALORIES	CARBS	PROTEIN	FAT	SODIUM
	g	g	g	g	g
Time	g	g	g	g	g
:	g	g	g	g	g
	g	g	g	g	g

Total

Friday _____   Month___   YR___

MEAL 1	CALORIES	CARBS	PROTEIN	FAT	SODIUM
	g	g	g	g	g
Time	g	g	g	g	g
:	g	g	g	g	g
	g	g	g	g	g

Total

MEAL 2	CALORIES	CARBS	PROTEIN	FAT	SODIUM
	g	g	g	g	g
Time	g	g	g	g	g
:	g	g	g	g	g
	g	g	g	g	g

Total

MEAL 3	CALORIES	CARBS	PROTEIN	FAT	SODIUM
	g	g	g	g	g
Time	g	g	g	g	g
:	g	g	g	g	g
	g	g	g	g	g

Total

MEAL 4	CALORIES	CARBS	PROTEIN	FAT	SODIUM
	g	g	g	g	g
Time	g	g	g	g	g
:	g	g	g	g	g
	g	g	g	g	g

Total

MEAL 5	CALORIES	CARBS	PROTEIN	FAT	SODIUM
	g	g	g	g	g
Time	g	g	g	g	g
:	g	g	g	g	g
	g	g	g	g	g

Total

Saturday _____   Month___   YR___

MEAL 1	CALORIES	CARBS	PROTEIN	FAT	SODIUM
	g	g	g	g	g
Time	g	g	g	g	g
:	g	g	g	g	g
	g	g	g	g	g

Total

MEAL 2	CALORIES	CARBS	PROTEIN	FAT	SODIUM
	g	g	g	g	g
Time	g	g	g	g	g
:	g	g	g	g	g
	g	g	g	g	g

Total

MEAL 3	CALORIES	CARBS	PROTEIN	FAT	SODIUM
	g	g	g	g	g
Time	g	g	g	g	g
:	g	g	g	g	g
	g	g	g	g	g

Total

MEAL 4	CALORIES	CARBS	PROTEIN	FAT	SODIUM
	g	g	g	g	g
Time	g	g	g	g	g
:	g	g	g	g	g
	g	g	g	g	g

Total

MEAL 5	CALORIES	CARBS	PROTEIN	FAT	SODIUM
	g	g	g	g	g
Time	g	g	g	g	g
:	g	g	g	g	g
	g	g	g	g	g

Total

Notes

Measurements

Neck   _____

Arms   _____

Chest   _____

Waist   _____

Hips   _____

Thighs   _____

Calves   _____

Weight   _____